Apprentice
in Black Stockings

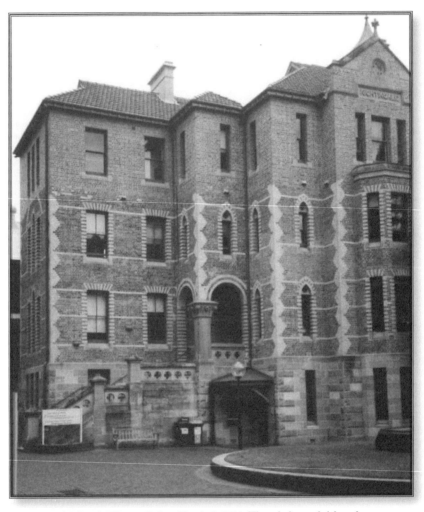

Nightingale Wing at Sydney Hospital, 2008. The polychrome brickwork was revealed after restoration in the 1990s.
(Author photograph)

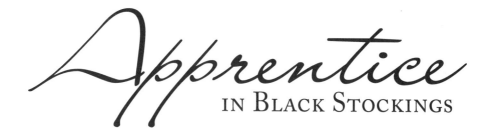
IN BLACK STOCKINGS

*An Australian
nursing memoir*

NORMA SIM

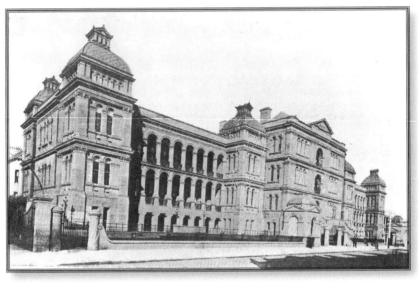

Sydney Hospital, 1911. (Courtesy of Sydney Hospital Medical Library)

*This book is dedicated
to Sydney Hospital
Nursing Trainees
1868–1984
and is a celebration
of the 220th Anniversary
of Sydney Hospital's Foundation*

Contents

Preface	9
Acknowledgments	11
Introduction: The Pioneering Days	13
1. The Apprentice	18
Uniform	27
Another Room	41
2. The Dumbstruck Patient	44
Fever	47
3. The Wintry Sea	52
Perfection	61
Dilemma	68
4. Social Intercourse	72
Relationships	73
Social Graces	87
5. Inner-city Life	93
6. Christmas Play	99
7. New Year, New Decade	104
8. Toil By Torchlight	110
Nightfall	116
9. The Straw and the Camel's Back	120
10. Back on Course	130
11. I Know Where I'm Going	136
12. Surreal Nights	142
13. The Virgins' Retreat	147

14. A Grim Revelation	151
15. Two City Shootings and an Explosion	157
Calamity	159
16. Surprises Prompt Contrasting Emotions	166
17. In the Land of Nod and Bedlam	175
18. Routines, Comparisons and the Unthinkable	181
19. Your Place or Mine	190
20. Broken Bones and Dented Dignity	193
Another thorn in the side	201
21. Milestones Celebrated	203
22. The Other Planet	211
Reflections	222
23. An End and a Beginning	227
Epilogue	231
Bibliography	237

Preface

Apprentice in Black Stockings is a memoir of a four-year period in my life in which I trained as a nurse at Sydney Hospital 60 years ago from 1949 to 1953.

Nursing is not an easy career path to pursue. Although it entails long hours and shift work, and is physically and emotionally testing, it is, however, always rewarding and a lesson in life's realities. Now that a university degree has replaced the old-style apprenticeship training, I felt it was important to capture the experiences from that earlier period. I hope my contribution assists in filling the gap in the genre of nursing memoir.

Sydney Hospital was the first hospital erected in Australia, functioning from 1788 to 1984 when the last group of trainee nurses graduated. Today, a small casualty department and Sydney Hospital remain at the rear of the building. The buildings of High Victoria architecture facing Macquarie Street, listed by the National Trust, are now utilised as government offices.

I have interspersed my own experiences with sections that describe nursing in the latter half of the nineteenth century at the time of Lucy Osburn and her five Nightingale nurses (they had been recruited by Florence Nightingale). Osburn and her small band of nurses arrived in the colony in 1868 to revolutionise the appalling nursing practices at Sydney Hospital and to initiate a training school for nurses, which had been non-existent until then. These sections on the Lucy Osburn days are in a different typeface from those relating to my own experiences of the 1950s. Though 80 years separate the two periods, very little had changed in nursing practice during that time. The Osburn scenes are based on fact but I have presented them as I imagine they might have been played out.

I have described the pleasures of living in the heart of the city, the importance of leisure time, and the social happenings that paved the way for a life after training against the backdrop of Sydney in the 1950s.

At the completion of my training in 1953, I married. I looked forward to my role as wife and mother, and thought I may not practice nursing again, but I was widowed three years later when I was eight months pregnant. Nursing was an ideal occupation to return to. I was left in a position that enabled me with a friend to purchase a 36-bed nursing home. I lived in as matron and kept my daughter with me. Later I worked part-time in various large Sydney hospitals and then became the manager of a medical bookshop until I retired. Writing, studying art history and literature are the rewards of this period.

Norma Sim

Acknowledgments

My grateful thanks to Bobbie Fookes. Without her support and computer skills this book would not have made the transition from memory onto the printed page.

I wish to acknowledge the assistance and information gained from Judith Godden's extensive biography, *Lucy Osburn: a lady displaced: Florence Nightingale's envoy to Australia*, which I have freely used as a source work when comparing the training at Sydney Hospital between 1949 and 1953 with Sydney Hospital of the second half of the nineteenth century. The anecdotes chosen from that earlier period, placed in juxtaposition with events I experienced, in some cases show things hadn't changed very much in 80 years. My versions of Lucy Osburn's era have been written as I imagine they might have been played out.

Thank you to David Todd for information supplied on some Sydney Hospital history. His great-grandmother, Nathalie Marx, was one of the first colonial nurses recruited to train under Miss Osburn and her Nightingale Nurses.

Thanks to New Holland Publishers and the staff involved in the production of this book.

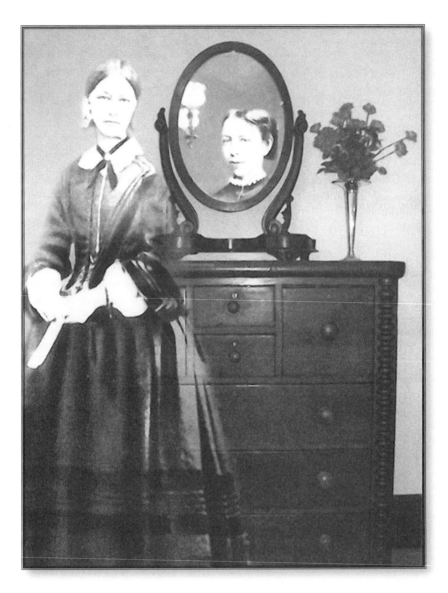

*Matron's dressing table and toilet mirror, circa 1868, showing an image of Florence Nightingale on the left and Lucy Osburn on the right.
(Courtesy of Lucy Osburn/Nightingale Museum, Sydney Hospital, Elinor Wrobel OAM, Curator)*

Introduction

The Pioneering Days

Sydney Hospital originated in a ship's hold, stowed aboard a vessel of the First Fleet sailing into Port Jackson in 1788. Part of the ship's cargo consisted of canvas and timber to be used for the specific purpose of erecting 'tent hospitals' for the sick convicts and free settlers. These tents were set up on the western side of Sydney Cove. Each one was shared by four patients lying on beds of grass or straw. One surgeon had been assigned to each of the 11 ships in the First Fleet and they all remained as medical staff in the new colony. Nursing was carried out by untrained, unpaid convicts.

The Second Fleet, which arrived in 1790, carried a prefabricated building made of 602 pieces of wood and copper, plus 100 tents to cope with overflow. The building was positioned near the present Overseas Terminal. The three ships of the Second Fleet brought more convicts, but 267 of them died on voyage, and 486 of those who survived the journey were sick or dying, bringing an influx of patients as well as building materials for an extended hospital to cope with the extra new settlers and convicts.

In 1796 the hospital was moved to a site near the Argyle Cut in The Rocks and re-erected on stone foundations.

In 1811 a new site was chosen for the hospital, which would become known as the Rum Hospital, on a 7-acre (nearly 3-hectare) elevated *prime site. The hospital was built by two prominent businessmen and would-be building contractors, Alexander Riley and Garnham Blaxcell. They secured this contract by applying to an advertisement in the* Sydney Gazette, *calling for tenders to build a general hospital, signed by D'Arcy Wentworth, Acting Principal Surgeon. Their knowledge of the rum trade was extensive, but they had no understanding of hospital construction. A street was formed to service the hospital and named Macquarie Street by Governor Lachlan Macquarie.*

In March 1868, Lucy Osburn arrived in the colony to take up her position as Lady Superintendent of Nursing at Sydney Hospital, or Sydney Infirmary as it was then known. This reform in colonial nursing had been instigated by politician Sir Henry Parkes and organised under Florence Nightingale's supervision. Miss Osburn found conditions similar to those in the convict era, incompetent nursing practised in filthy surroundings. A pardoned convict and former matron, Mrs Bethsheba Ghost, had left just two years before Lucy Osburn's arrival. The hospital was staffed with nursing personnel made up of men and women, all untrained. They worked 15-hour shifts, from 6 in the morning until 9 at night when the wards would be locked and a wardsman, usually an ex-patient, slept in a room adjacent to the ward. Miss Osburn's formidable task was to implement an efficient professional nursing system and to replace the dysfunctional unhygienic practices then in place.

In 1881 the 1811 building was demolished. It had become filled with vermin and 60 years of accumulated filth in the drainage system due to its disgraceful construction.

In 1894 a new 315-bed hospital was completed with some delay because of ballooning costs and the architect, Thomas Rowe, being replaced. The new architect was John Kirkpatrick. The present-day State Parliament and the Mint buildings were originally part of the hospital, giving both the hospital and Macquarie Street a grand style. These two were handed over to their later uses in 1829 and 1855 respectively.

Miss Osburn and her five nurses sailed to Australia aboard Dunbar Castle via the Cape of Good Hope, a non-stop journey of three months.

Miss Osburn travelled first class, but the five nurses were allotted cramped conditions in facilities provided for Female Servants of First Class Passengers. They were under Miss Osburn's supervision but the obvious differences in class accommodation caused some resentment.

This arrangement may have set a precedent in the association between Head of Nursing and her nurses for decades to come in the colony. All six women had undergone one year of training under Matron Wardroper in the Nightingale School of Nursing at St Thomas's Hospital, London and had gained varying terms of experience in nursing before or after training except for one woman, Haldane Turriff.

Miss Nightingale was strong in her assessment of the qualities her nurses must have. It was essential that 'she be a "gentlewoman", punctual, quiet, trustworthy, neat and clean'. Hygiene was to be of utmost importance during all nursing practices. She was impressed with Lucy Osburn and the five nurses selected by Miss Wardroper as they set out on their mission to revolutionise nursing in Sydney. She compared them with the 38 nurses she had taken out to Scutari during the Crimean War in 1854, describing that group, faced with caring for horrific war casualties, as:

> Poor drinking rabble ... with the feckless, ignorant, romantic ladies ... with the six nurses of St John's House, the six most perfectly useless specimens of the animal creation I have ever seen ... with the eight ceremonial twaddlers belonging to Miss Sellon ... with the converting childish fools of nuns ... whom I took out.
> (A letter from Floernce Nightingale to Henry Bonham Carter, 2 December 1868, in Godden, page 77)

The five Nightingales Lucy Osburn brought to the colony were Mary

Barker, Eliza Blundell, Bessie Chant, Annie Miller and Haldane Colquhoun Turriff.

Mary Barker, was 39 years old, very religious and the least educated of the group. She was respectable, but had a temper. It was said that, while she may not treat her patients tenderly, she would never neglect them.

Eliza Blundell, a 28-year-old widow, was attentive to her duties, a good practical nurse, impulsive and sometimes noisy, and pretty.

Bessie Chant, 30 years old, was good, plain, intelligent, amiable and kind—the one without any peculiarities of temper.

Annie Miller, 34 years old, was respectable, proud and peculiarly sensitive. When Florence Nightingale interviewed Annie, she noted with disapproval that Annie and Bessie Chant had each worn a large black buckle and brooch on their uniforms, which should have been devoid of decoration.

Haldane Colquhoun Turriff, 33 years old, was intelligent, with superior abilities and education. She was described as a shrewd, clever Scotswoman of haughty spirit, capable of displaying a violent temper, and inclined to write mischievous letters to other nurses during her training.

Miss Wardroper was sure Miss Osburn would exercise her power of control. The truth was Lucy Osburn had no real experience in managing staff.

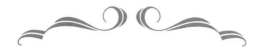

Twelve Indispensable Qualities Desirable in the Nurse

1. *Orderliness*
2. *Deportment*
3. *Truthfulness*
4. *Loyalty*
5. *Accuracy*
6. *Cleanliness*
7. *Sympathy, Tact and Understanding*
8. *Economy*
9. *Reliability*
10. *Obedience*
11. *Observation*
12. *Punctuality*

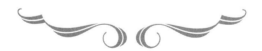

I

The Apprentice

17 October 1949

There is no pulling back now or initiating a cowardly change of heart by retracing my steps down Martin Place.

I fidget nervously while balancing on the kerb's edge. The traffic lights have alerted pedestrians to 'cross now'.

The flowing sea of Macquarie Street motor vehicles is stemmed and, like the parting of waters, allows a crossing into a land largely unknown to me. Entry into the hospital grounds is through permanently open wrought-iron gates, fronting a facade of High Victorian architecture at once imposing but faintly grim. A structure of Sydney sandstone fits formally into the landscape of the top end of Martin Place.

Two three-storey ward pavilions are graced with rhythmically arcaded stone verandas, filled in with ornate cast iron and timber balustrades. Both are linked to the middle administration building by arched stone bridges. Early morning shadows slowly melt into soft gold as increasing sunlight seeps into the sandstone, lessening the structure's forbidding aspect.

The suitcase handle is clutched firmly in my hand as I quicken my steps, passing the gatekeeper wedged into the doorway of his gatehouse, a sandstone construction in miniature. The driveway accommodates pedestrians and ambulances alike, then widens out into a grass-covered courtyard.

Water drizzles quietly over a black cast-iron fountain, flowing through a nest of swans then down to a circle of cranes, their flight frozen in metal. Folded wings glisten and clawed feet are bathed before the water is finally meted out in a mild circular disturbance on the surrounding pool.

The wide stone staircase of the Nightingale Wing is a few steps away.

An earlier decision has brought me here on 17 October 1949, shortly before my nineteenth birthday. It was shaped by the interference of war and was compounded by the shock announcement that my mother, after 15 years, had fallen pregnant, giving birth to her second daughter—an event which was to occupy her full attention and coincide with the year of my leaving school at Intermediate Certificate level.

The first shell fired in the submarine attack on Sydney Harbour in 1942 had put paid to my filling the place reserved for me at a city boarding school to study for the Leaving Certificate, which was not available in our small country town. This narrowed my career choices considerably.

Fate steered me in another direction. I had come across an article in an old *Pix* magazine, a picture-story depicting the training of a nurse at Sydney Hospital. Nursing seemed a noble profession, one filled with smiling young women, and importantly would offer a chance to live in the city with pay and the provision of accommodation.

With one gloved hand I press the button circled in shining brass.

Fate has set the course and raised a wind to fill the sails. I draw in a deep breath, uncertain of a smooth passage ahead but buoyed by a sudden feeling of optimism.

A bell resounds within the building; footsteps clop on highly polished linoleum; and a bustling elderly maid clothed in a brown uniform and covering white apron emerges out of a shadowy recess, a corridor faintly lit beneath a frugal light bulb. The tiny woman has little to say, just a few words which direct me to enter and turn towards the Visitors' Sitting Room. Then she darts away, vanishing down the gloomy corridor on her thin, quick legs. A shaft of sunlight streams through the glass panes set in french doors at the end. I can see sun-dappled treetops in the bordering Domain swaying in a nor'easter that is already building up off the harbour.

I wonder why the maid turns on her heel and departs so swiftly, not knowing she has many duties to carry out, and the irritating doorbell, which rings many more times this morning, will interfere with her schedule.

In the following weeks I will notice her bustling about, filling in a long day, devoted to Matron and seeing to her needs, making certain she is not distracted from official duties by the mundane domestic chores of everyday existence. These include cleaning Matron's private accommodation, with its extensive views out over the Botanic Gardens and harbour, serving her meals in the dining room behind her office and checking her laundry, ensuring her impeccable presentation in white starched uniform, veil, stockings and shoes freshly coated in white Kiwi paint.

I had seen Matron when I was interviewed several months earlier. Colour is not associated with Matron Elsie Pidgeon. Her pale, powdered complexion, a rebellious wisp of wayward grey hair which dares to escape from under her veil, leaves her an unmistakable vision in white and denotes her singular superior position.

Directly opposite the vestibule I pass the door to Matron's office, which stands ajar and Miss Osburn's photograph is revealed, hanging on the far wall. She had posed for the camera while seated and appears thoughtful, allowing the faint glimmer of a smile to appear. Resting her elbow on several books she gives the impression of one with a studious mind, as no doubt this prop was meant to convey. Her dress, made up in a heavy dark material imparts a soft sheen, and an austere muslin headpiece falls from hair parted in the middle and hangs down past her shoulder. Miss Osburn's portrait will become more familiar to me on future visits to Matron's office.

Before entering the Visitors' Sitting Room I pass another open doorway that leads into a spacious room, filled to the brim with young women dressed in uniform. A buzz of words and laughter drifts out into the hallway, riding on the acrid smell of cigarette smoke and I think how pleasant it would be to pull the pack from my handbag, light up and soothe my fluttering nerves. The Visitors' Sitting Room is a smaller, sedate room with a marble fireplace obviously unlit in this century. By way of an apology for this neglect, the grate is filled with tired, dried-out pine cones. Ponderous Victorian furniture overfills the room.

Seated on a chaise longue is a lone girl, the first of nine to arrive.

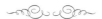

The October day continues under balmy sunshine as I view my surroundings from a firstfloor bedroom window in the Nightingale Wing.

Groups of pigeons quarrel and flutter along the eaves of the nearby hospital wing. Some balance higher up clinging to a miniature Roman temple that crowns a green cupola clad in fish-scale copper shingles—an unexpected Italianate influence at each corner of the north and south buildings.

My eyes travel downwards from the roof to a ward veranda, fenced in with wire, which overlooks the courtyard and I can see a line of patients lying in beds placed against the wall.

The pathways that surround the central courtyard are busy with people entering or leaving the grounds, seeking out wards, departments, casualty and other tucked-away areas. The higher walkways between adjoining buildings are occasionally enlivened by the passing motion of a white veil or doctor's coat. The prospect of joining their ranks instils a brief twinge of nervous excitement.

Turning away to face my allotted bed, I survey the room shared with three of the eight other probationers who, one by one, had been shown into the sitting room downstairs, introduced themselves to each other, then, seated stiffly, eyed one another tentatively.

If a prize were to be offered for the most bleak and uninviting room one might live in this must win. It has a decor of brown linoleum, brown blinds, brown furniture and lacks curtains, heating or ornamentation.

I have a magpie need for shiny colour and to my mind, in a world where delightful colours of the spectrum can be appreciated, mixed or blended, the colour brown, if indeed it is a colour, must be the most unattractive. For a moment I think of my bedroom at home, a long distance away on the far North Coast, decorated by my mother's skill in pinks and green.

Quickly brought back into the present by my chattering room-mates, now bright and friendly and expressing some of the apprehension I feel, we are the most junior of junior nursing personnel. We will remain probationers in an apprenticeship for the first year, gradually moving up the ladder with the next intake of Tutor School students.

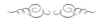

My unwilling fingers fumble with the back tab on my suspender belt. The thickness of black stocking resists fitting between the rubber tab and the metal clip; stockings that I purchased as listed on the sheet of requirements: 'must be opaque so that no skin is visible underneath'. This causes some giggling as we change into uniforms selected from the stack placed on each bed. A week's supply of dresses, aprons and various starched accessories as yet to be identified.

'No doubt the thickness of stocking has been stipulated in order to prevent male patients fantasising over our hidden flesh,' is Janet's assumption, said with a twinkle in her eye. I think she is very pretty and admire her soft voice and mannered body language.

At this moment there is a knock and a head appears around the door.

'Need any help with the uniform?' a cheerful voice enquires.

'Come in, come in,' we chorus our answer.

By the time our visitor arrives we have reached the stage of applying the outer highly starched layer that covers a blue and white dress.

'Sister Breakall asked me to see if you need assistance.' The helpful nurse, who is wearing a probationers' cap, glances at her watch pulled out from the breast pocket behind her apron bib.

'It won't do to keep her waiting.' Then adding, 'Although she's not one of the fiery ones.'

We four novices look questioningly at each other. The expression on everyone's face seems to indicate we must all be thinking: 'What does she mean by fiery?' No-one queries this, as it seems we are expected to know.

The helpful nurse places the snow-white apron around my waist—one edge folds over the other at the back and is secured with a safety pin. The bib covers the chest, wide straps continue over the shoulders and crisscross then are pinned at the waist. A collar, cardboard stiff, is placed around the neck, secured with a stud; the cap worn in first year must hide all hair at the back, caught up and tucked underneath the muslin. A small peak is fashioned in the band above each ear. Long sleeves are covered at the wrist by

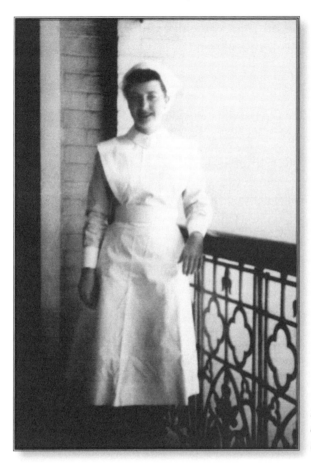

17 October 1949, author on first day of training. (Author photograph)

added starched cuffs and a starched belt circles the waist, buttoned with two studs. Walking towards a full-length mirror attached to the back of my wardrobe door the starched apron feels and moves like large sheets of newspaper around my legs, my image is a replica of the nurse in the *Pix* article. The transformation causes a few 'Nightingale' twinges within my chest.

Someone on the far side of the room is looking into her mirror vigorously trying to tuck an unruly head of hair into her cap and gives her opinion. 'I look and feel like a milkmaid,' followed by a nervous giggle.

Each girl has been fitted for uniforms during an appointment made with the hospital's dressmaker in Paddington. The

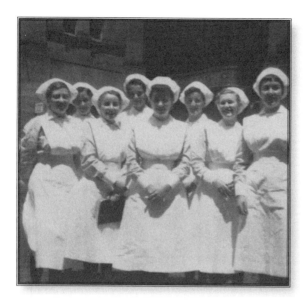

The group of new recruits on the first day, 17 October 1949. (Author photograph)

dressmaker works from home, a tiny nineteenth-century terrace, a one-storey design multiplied to make a row named Rose Terrace. Pedalling rapidly on her Singer sewing machine as though to keep afloat in a sea of blue and white yardage, plain blue wool for capes, spools of white and blue cotton, the scattered bolts of material look like logs floating around her. A short visit to the city several weeks earlier was necessary to attend this fitting and undergo a medical examination.

The result of that visit to Rose Terrace brings us to our dress rehearsal. The stage manager, Sister Lyle Breakall, is waiting on the podium for our first performance, the presentation of her new Tutor School group. We must appear punctually on cue.

We gather together in the hallway. Shod in brand new black shoes made by 'Mr Hall', possibly somewhere in a Redfern footwear factory, we negotiate the spiral stairway leading down to the next floor.

Passing by Matron's open office door my sensible lace-ups are squeaking loudly.

I make a mental note to wet the soles tonight and stuff them with newspaper. A sure remedy for the protestations of new leather.

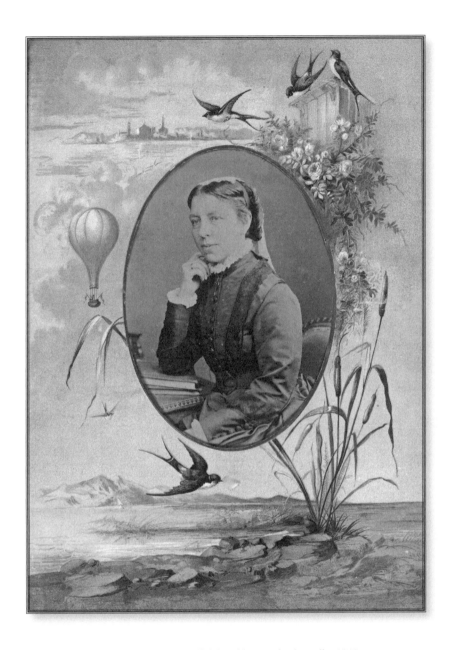

*Lucy Osborn, Florence Nightingale's envoy in Australia, 1868.
(Courtesy of Mitchell Library, State Library of NSW, Call Number: PXA345)*

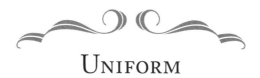

Uniform

Uniform is to be worn ... daily in or out of the Infirmary boundary by the five Nightingale nurses who accompany Miss Osburn. Their everyday uniforms designed for wearing in Sydney are approved by Miss Wardroper and Miss Nightingale, measured and made up in a pale grey fabric in St Thomas's sewing room.

Nearing completion of the year's training and with their sailing date drawing closer, the Sisters wait to view the completed 'walking out' uniform.

Moving across the room, Eliza Blundell pauses by the window. Steely grey clouds are low over the city and a miserly sleet is feathering down, laying a treacherous coating over the cobblestones. Slipping horse hooves and hoarse cries of coachmen berating their animals can be heard.

Inside, the atmosphere of the sitting room is quiet. The occasional shifting of coals in the fireplace and scant conversation break the silence. Some speculation is voiced about the coming sea voyage and the expectation of a warmer climate at journey's end, with bleak days like this left behind.

Miss Osburn enters the room, followed by the seamstress and her assistant, arms wrapped around bundles of uniforms and caps. These are laid out over the centre table while Miss Osburn stands on the other side.

Newly designed in preparation for Sydney and for wearing when outside the Infirmary precincts, the garments are now revealed. The Sisters have already voiced disapproval on consideration of the cap to be worn while on duty, regarding it as an adornment usually worn by trainees or older women. Now they express the desire to wear their own apparel when going out.

'Where is your pride in the uniform?' is Lucy's lament. 'Can you not take a nobler attitude and think less of fashionable dresses and shawls?'

She surveys her personal choice of working attire laid across the sofa back. It is appropriate in her position as head of the Nightingale nurses to wear a different style to those the nurses are viewing. Her selection is a floor-length woollen dress in black, bound to draw the heat in a Sydney summer and no doubt the fabric will have to be modified for later outfits. The heaviness of tone is relieved by white linen collar and cuffs, and a white muslin bonnet.

Eliza Blundell speaks out, with a complaint quickly taken up by her fellow nurses.

'So drab. We will be inconspicuous in a dress of such dullness. Who will recognise our position or care to admire our appearance?' Eliza always liked to be noticed, responding by preening with a smoothing of her hair and drawing up of her small frame.

'Brown dress, black cloak and the white straw of the bonnet covered by a black veil.' She bluntly describes the outfit aware that it will not draw complimentary remarks.

Miss Osburn releases a long sigh. 'This has Miss Nightingale's approval and therefore no more can be said.'

However, she appears to be giving further consideration to the subject. Eliza would like to point out a few facts but hesitates. What would Miss Nightingale know about going out? She has become an invalid by confining herself to bed for the past 11 years since 1857. Better not to voice these thoughts. Eliza waits for Lucy's reply to her complaint. Miss Osburn fingers the dark brown material and makes a small concession.

'When we reach our destination perhaps the bonnet trimming can be changed from brown to blue.'

She does not voice her true thoughts that, just as a nun is recognised by her black habit, an austere outdoor uniform will distinguish the Nightingale nurses and make them very careful and circumspect in their behaviour. She is already regretting her earlier lenience in proposing the change of colour for the bonnet ribbon.

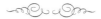

Pretty Eliza Blundell balances firmly on the rolling deck moving her weight from one small foot to the other. The group is well into this exciting adventure and Eliza is the one who intends to relish every moment. Looking upwards towards the poop deck, then higher into the swaying spars with one hand sheltering her eyes, she loves to watch the sailors at their work. More thrilling is the scene when, ceasing to strain on the ropes while the boatswain sings a line or two of his solo song then singing in unison, they pull together and the coordination of male muscles ripples with the effort. They are aware of Eliza's admiration as she smiles and waves. Miss Osburn is also aware and has taken steps to keep a watchful eye on her flirtatious protégée. She moves Eliza out of the cabin she shares with her fellow nurses and into Lucy's own cabin so she can monitor Eliza's movements more closely.

At the close of the tedious three-month voyage to the opposite end of the globe, the Dunbar Castle slips in, riding a fair onshore wind through the jagged portals guarding Port Jackson. It is the end of the nurses' first venture abroad.

Miss Osburn is a more experienced traveller, having visited Europe and Palestine. She is glad to see the last of the seven other passengers on board, none of whom had impressed her as travelling companions. The nurses are rowed ashore, eagerly anticipating stepping onto dry land again, as there had been no ports of call on the way.

Waiting for them on the wharf is the statesman Sir Henry Parkes. His stolid figure, wealth of white beard and head crowned with a black top hat stands out as he moves forward to greet the women warmly. Miss Osburn introduces her nurses. Each one referred to as Sister, followed by their Christian name, a title chosen by Florence Nightingale, which, she was quick to reassure her critics, had no religious connotations.

Arriving at the Infirmary gates, stepping down from the horse-drawn carriage onto the Macquarie Street pavement, she is welcomed by Mrs Cole, the retiring Housekeeper-Matron. Lucy is surprised and pleased with the town's appearance and the Infirmary's elegant facade. Before following on the heels of the nervous little housekeeper, she casts her eyes up to the veranda running the length of the building. Several sets of curious eyes are summing up the new Lady Superintendent.

John Blackstone is one watching the arrival of this new threat to his role as manager. A fine-looking woman, he must admit. They could work together as long as she doesn't interfere in his position. There is a nasty streak in Blackstone's character: Miss Osburn should watch her step.

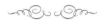

Carrying out her inspection the following day, Miss Osburn is appalled to discover that the hospital's grand exterior belies the state of the interior. Whatever her expectations, she is not prepared for the disorder and filth that abound.

On completing this appraisal, Miss Osburn takes a short rest in a deep chair placed in the sitting room provided for her. Head propped against the padded headrest, she can barely keep her eyes open. Sleep had evaded her the previous night. The day is hotter than usual for early autumn and, reminding herself to change out of her 'uniform', the heavy woollen dress, into her black silk for the coming afternoon, she listens to the sounds filtering through her fitful dozing.

The outside courtyard is filled with a harsh light that hurts the eyes, as she had discovered on venturing out that morning on an inspection of various outbuildings. Someone out there in the heat is giving an order in a raised voice. Lucy stirs as a carriage rattles over the courtyard flagstones. The clip-clop of horses' hooves and jingling harness cause memories of London streets to surface.

Suddenly, startled, her eyes fly open with the awareness someone has entered the room, and she is immediately annoyed to see Sister Haldane Turriff easing herself down into the adjacent chair, settling her upper limbs along the padded armrests and stretching her legs. Sister Haldane is a shrewd and mischievous woman, with a penchant for eavesdropping on her fellow Sisters, while reporting her version of events in a private correspondence to Florence Nightingale. Already she and Sister Annie Miller, her fellow Scotswoman, have developed an intense dislike for each other. Lucy suspects this visit is another attempt to ingratiate herself with her Lady Superintendent.

'What are your impressions of these colonial nurses, Miss Osburn? Have you in all your life seen such a raw lot? And attired like slum dwellers.'

While Lucy struggles to bring her mind into focus, Haldane elaborates on her description. 'A rough group they are indeed ... no conformity in dress or colour, worn and ragged clothing, no aprons and no caps so that their greasy unkempt hair is hanging loose about their shoulders!'

Lucy is deliberating on her own description to be penned to Miss Nightingale and will do so later, writing in all truth: 'The present nurses are as rough and callow a group as I have seen, obviously brought up in hugger-mugger Irish ways without a clear or systematic idea in their heads.'

Yes, she is thinking, there is no other way I can describe them to Miss Nightingale and, then turning to Haldane, reveals how she might begin to tackle the task ahead.

'I hope to be able to choose a few, perhaps three, of the existing nurses, if they are suitable, and invite applicants in the colony to be interviewed and selected to train under us.'

The subject of uniform is raised once more. 'These trainees should wear a lilac uniform, white apron and goffered frill cap tied under the chin. Moving throughout the ward, when clean and in order, fulfilling their duties, they will bring some cheer to the scene.' There is a pause as Miss Osburn paints this picture in her mind, then adding, 'like moving components of colour'.

Sister Haldane raises her eyebrows, draws in a loud sniff through her nose. Satisfied with the Sisters' indoor uniform, which envelops her *rigid form in pale grey, she is by no means a colourful person, but an all-round grey person, with a sallow skin, severe expression and with no desire to pay attention to fripperies.*

A balmy breeze is picking up, strengthening as it travels up the slope from harbour to town and entering the open window. It does nothing to dispel the unsavoury odour emanating from the nearby ward. Rising to her feet, feeling a little more refreshed after her brief nap, Miss Osburn dismisses Sister Haldane and moves to prepare herself before meeting with those scheduled to make her acquaintance in the afternoon hours.

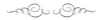

Sister Lyle Breakall, our Tutor Sister for the next six weeks, is taking us on a tour of the hospital.

I regard Lyle as a male name, having known only one other christened as such, a boy, briefly a boyfriend. He was handsome, with a fresh rose flush on the fine skin of each cheek and a personality that emphasised his good looks.

His sexiness must have also registered with my mother. She would call me in if she thought our goodnights extended too long as we stood at the front door adjacent to her bedroom window. He joined the navy soon after, and I was spared any further embarrassment of being summoned inside.

My oscillating mind, moved by a name, swings back and remains anchored. I concentrate on Sister Breakall. She is quite small, fortyish, with an attractive face and china blue eyes. She is turned out in the Sisters' uniform as neatly as anyone could be: a French blue with two perpendicular rows of white buttons down the front, large V-shaped white collar, cuffs, stockings and shoes. A perfectly starched muslin veil covers her hair and, folded in a triangular shape, its wide wings float out over her shoulders. She must have come off duty at some time in her training with a soiled apron, cap askew and perhaps a piece of patient's food riding on her shoe, but it is hard to imagine. She reminds me of a small doll I once busily cared for as a child, diligently laundering and pressing her outfit before standing her up in front of admiring playmates.

We are a captive group clustered in our tutor's wake. We follow her white veil as though it represents a symbol of security, and she leads the way across the courtyard and into an entrance at the base of a building facing Macquarie Street. An unfamiliar odour permeates the air, a mixture of cleaning agents, antiseptics and other unknown quantities that hangs in the corridors of all buildings where the sick are treated. As time passes, this smell will become unnoticeable to me.

The starched apron is too tight across my thighs, a weakness is felt in my knees, the starched belt is constricting and my head begins to ache. This is the first day of my menstrual period, always problematic, with pain and a dragging down sensation in my lower abdomen. I wish I could lie down on my side somewhere and pull my knees up. I am unaware at this time that an analgesic medication for this problem can be obtained at Matron's office. The tour of orientation continues, up wide and splendid cedar staircases, across adjoining covered passageways, under lofty pressed tin ceilings, until we pause before double blue-grey painted doors with etched glass panels, hinged back onto brass floor catches.

This is our first viewing of a ward.

All the wards, with the exception of Ward I, are set up as Nightingale wards in dormitory style. This one has a row of possibly seven beds down each side and four across the far end wall—Florence approved of the open vista enabling the staff to have all patients in their view.

We bypass the lofty vestibule of the impressive front entrance, skirt wards, using their verandas as passageways, moving up or down a ramp here and there with seemingly no order in the layout. The 1894 Worrall Theatre was designed by architect John Kirkpatrick. The eastern wall is curved and the outside is accentuated by a turret capped with a witch's hat slate roof placed at each end. This gives the exterior architecture a fairytale appearance. The starkness of the wall's interior is relieved by two circular stained-glass windows.

There are odours of a different kind lurking in this area. My previous experience of hospital smells and sounds had occurred before a tonsillectomy performed in my hometown hospital's operating theatre when I was 17 years old.

I recalled the stench of ether dripped onto a facial mask enclosing mouth and nose. The sound of someone's voice instructing me to breathe in, as I fought to rip off the smothering device.

The next visit to that stark room came after scrambling up an oyster-encrusted pole, part of the fencing in the local seaside pool. The razor cut from a jagged oyster shell became infected; it was necessary to lance the toe, which was swollen with grey pus and had taken on the appearance of the plump oyster that was once the shell's tenant.

White-clad figures, nose, mouth and hair hidden, hurry by our group, which is gathered around Sister Breakall in the theatre's anteroom. We do our best to appear nonchalant. A difficult pose when forced to stand, hands behind backs, concentrating on Sister's words.

Our peaked caps, newly stiff with the first wearing and steeped in starch, are a tell-tale sign, as a flag on a tall mast identifies a ship.

The Renwick Pavilion, built in 1907, the Kanematsu Memorial Institute, built in 1933, the wards, Want Theatre and lecture hall, the 1930 Travers Building with wards, Casualty, Maitland Theatre and nurses' sick bay all mix in my mind, along with many other departments, Outpatients, X-Ray, Pharmacy and the Chapel. Finally we are heading back towards the Nightingale Wing.

My stomach is a hollow cavern rumbling in protest at my neglect of its needs.

'You may take an hour for lunch today,' Sister Breakall checks her watch. 'Be in the Tutor School by 1.30.' We follow her towards the dining room, situated on the ground floor below the main entrance to the Nightingale Wing.

The dining room is almost filled with nursing staff, the hum of conversation hangs in the air. A maid points to a vacant table, pausing in her delivery of meals. Pulling out chairs, we seat ourselves and, as one, sigh and look at each other. Janet is the first to speak. We will learn that she is the one who will always be full of optimism.

'That was all very interesting, don't you think?' Her smile reveals perfect teeth, and her large brown eyes twinkle. 'I'm sure

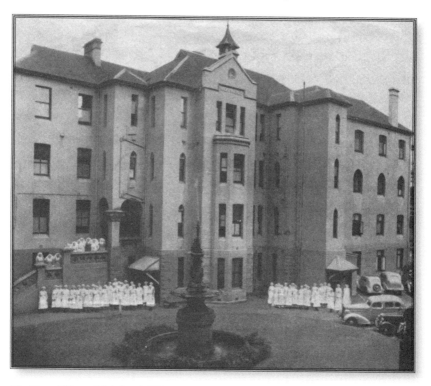

The Nurses' Home, Nightingale Wing, at Sydney Hospital, circa 1950. (Courtesy of Sydney Hospital Medical Library)

we will all fit in very well.' With no response and everyone rather subdued, she hurries on. 'I'm starving. Does anyone else feel the same?'

Before anyone can reply there is a teeth-on-edge screech of chair legs scraping, cutlery dropping on crockery and everyone is standing, including those at the Sisters' table on the far side of the room. Our group follow suit, albeit a little more slowly. There is a hush. Matron Pidgeon has descended the staircase leading down from the floor above into the dining room's centre. She speaks briefly with one of the Sisters and, turning, ascends the stairs. The drone of conversation and the dining room clatter recommence, as though on cue. Janet is the first to make a comment.

'That must be a show of respect for her position. I suppose there are certain strict lines of protocol we must adhere to.'

'Sounds something like being in the army,' I reply, my eyes searching the dining room for some sign of an approaching dinner plate. 'What other regulations do you think will surprise us?' The abdominal cramps have settled, replaced by hunger pains.

'You will all know there is a curfew placed on the Nurses' Home?' Judy is the quiet one. A faint blush colours her complexion whenever she speaks in her slow country drawl, as though her adding to a conversation might be embarrassing for her. 'We have to be in by 11 p.m. every night.'

'Yes, but we are allowed one late pass per month,' Barbara adds. 'It is as though I am continuing on with boarding school.' She has an infectious laugh that is great to hear. She was last to arrive that morning, breathless, carrying a violin case, wearing gloves (always worn in the street as taught by the nuns and removed indoors). She seems the most delicate and ladylike—perhaps the one least likely to survive this career choice.

Pat is the next to speak in her assured voice, chin lifted and eyeing everyone in turn. She would keep us all amused with stagy antics in later dismal times. Pat was a former pupil in drama under

Doris Fitton at the Independent Theatre. We are impressed when she reveals this and, when asked why she hadn't carried on with acting, she replies, 'There is no money in that career, my dears, and precious little in this one.' Now she adds in answer to Barbara's remark on late passes, 'There is some leniency, the pass can be extended to 2.30 a.m. on special occasions.'

'What other restraints are placed upon us?' I speculate and June offers one more.

'We all know it's compulsory to live in,' and, perhaps because she is a few years older than most of us and could have matrimony on her mind, adds 'and I'm sure you must know marriage is forbidden during training.' The conversation turns away from rules and regulations and moves onto impressions gained from the hospital inspection just completed.

At last a maid is approaching with a tray and I remember my mother voicing some warnings as I compare the quality of food on the plate placed in front of me with her delicious cooking. She had pointed out some unpleasant tasks involved in nursing and the disadvantages of shift work. I was determined to prove my mother wrong. Shift work is no impediment when your social and love life are nought.

A roast dinner is on the menu today, an example of the meals that will follow seven days a week, 52 weeks a year over four years. We are not sure which beast has been slaughtered in order to end up on this table, whether lamb, beef or pork. The slices of meat are overcooked, with frayed edges curling up out of a pool of pale, cornflour gravy, and vegetables clearly baked over a long period, destroying any individual taste, avoiding the necessity to discard a particular one because we do not normally eat it. And where are the vases of flowers? The *Pix* photograph of the Nurses' Dining Room shows a vase of flowers on every table; long stemmed poppies supporting wide cheerful heads. I push the meat slices through the congealing gravy to one side of the plate and concentrate on the unidentifiable vegetables. A curdled baked milk pudding and tinned peaches follow.

'I have my camera upstairs.' Placing her cutlery down onto her plate, Pauline pushes her chair back. 'I'll run upstairs and get it. We must have a shot of us on this day, all together in front of the fountain. I'll meet you there.'

Pauline musters us into a line like a mother hen arranging the presentation of her chicks to the world. She is perhaps five years older and fills the role of mother perfectly. We pose self-consciously, myself in the centre, hands held together across my apron, everyone concentrating on the Box Brownie's lens.

Once again on this day, we are made painfully aware of our unmistakable 'newness' under the scrutiny of passing staff.

Entering the nurses' packed sitting room for the first time is also an ordeal, feeling all eyes must be on us. As we hover in the doorway there is a sudden spontaneous evacuation of the room; time for those on afternoon shift to move to their various wards. Some quickly descend the front entrance steps and scatter across the courtyard. Others smartly negotiate the iron spiral stairway with a ringing sound of black duty shoes hitting metal, down and out through the side exit on the ground floor. Our group take vacant chairs in one corner of the empty room opposite three phone booths situated on the far wall and Janet moves to make a call to her mother. How I would love to ring home, but to do that I will have to walk down Martin Place to the GPO, book a long distance call and wait. Eventually the switchboard operator will make the connection after working through her list of those waiting and my number will be called to summon me to an allocated phone booth. This will be my priority when I have the cash. Meanwhile I will write every week.

To hear my mother's voice at that moment may be overwhelming.

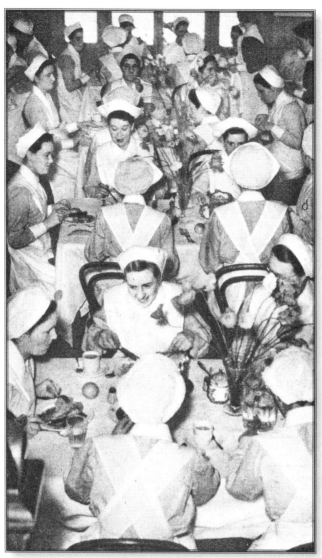

Nurses' Dining Room, Sydney Hospital, circa 1940.
*(*Pix *magazine, courtesy of Mitchell Library, State Library of NSW)*

The bed is neither comfortless nor comfortable, just unfamiliar. My head is filled with remembrances; a luscious roast leg of lamb sizzling in our kitchen stove on Sundays, juicy corn picked off stalks in my uncle's cornfield, the cobs' silk shimmering under the sun, flaky scones and steamed puddings so light there is no chewing required, all baked in my mother's kitchen.

Light patterns float across the ceiling from the headlights of an outward bound ambulance.

Gentle night sounds circle within the room. Soft breathing of someone in a deep sleep, the creaking of a bed; strangely comforting as I have never shared a room with anyone before.

Sporadic faint cooing from the roof pigeons drifts in. No members of this avian breed frequent my home town but they seem to cluster in droves in the public spaces and on the roofs around the city.

Sitting up I place my feet on the cool linoleum then move silently across the room careful not to wake the others. From the window I peep out. There are more unfamiliar sounds in the night; trickling water recycling a course throughout the fountain, the intermittent wail of a human voice persists for a time then ceases.

'What can you see?' whispers Judy raising her head, peering through the gloom.

'Very little,' I answer softly. 'Victorian architecture on all sides and here and there behind the ward blinds, a dim light'. A shadowy figure enters the scene and I report 'light from a torch moving along a veranda. Nothing much at all.' I wonder how it feels to be the lone nurse at night behind the blinds in that withdrawn world.

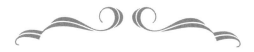

ANOTHER ROOM

Lesser creatures—largely intolerable ... is a mild description for intruders encountered by Lucy Osburn during her first night on colonial soil and the reason she missed her yearned for, refreshing, sleep.

The room Mrs Cole has prepared is a makeshift one. Plans for the Nightingale Wing, a separate building to house the nursing staff, have been appraised and approved by Miss Nightingale, but construction will not be completed until the following year, though those original plans will be framed and hung in Miss Osburn's office, and continue to be displayed through following decades.

Arrival in the new Colony is followed by a day filled with appointments and the shaking of many hands, including those of the 27 members of the Hospital Board. A quick inspection of the Infirmary layout, then onto Government House to lunch with the charming Lady Belmore, wife of the governor, Lord Belmore. Returning the short distance along Macquarie Street and meeting more visitors at the Infirmary continues until well past 9 p.m.

Lucy steps out of her black silk dress, slips on her nightgown, splashes her face with cool water poured from a jug into the washstand basin and turns the lamp down to burn on a low flame. The sparse circle of light glows faintly in the room. The ship still seems to move beneath her bare feet after three months at sea. To lie down and defeat that rocking sensation and get some rest is imperative.

Hospital sounds, though muffled, enter—raucous coughing, padding feet, a slamming door. The howl of a patient in pain, calling for attention and ignored until other plaintive cries join in, chorusing out of tune until finally lessening, perhaps with the arrival of a nurse, *awakened and disgruntled. The colonial nurses sleep in the wards behind screens, while in some wards doors are locked at 9 p.m. and patients rely on a wardsman, elderly and an ex-patient, who sleeps in an adjoining room, to tend to their needs. These sounds are not new to Lucy and merciful sleep soon envelops her tired body.*

Rest is short lived, dispersed by an itching, stinging sensation over most of her body and she is quickly awake and alert to the night's whispers, different to those that sent her drifting into sleep. Close to her bed, in the wall, rasping noises filter through the cracked plaster as multitudes of insects scramble over the crumbling internal brickwork. Several cockroaches, pearly black, the largest she has ever seen, emerge and, as fast as runaway horses, speed down the wall to the skirting board. The claws of a scuttling hairy creature scratch the bare floor. She is wide awake, turning up the bedside lamp in time to see a rat lurking in the corner, luminous eyes briefly mesmerised by the lamplight, the squeaking of metal bed springs sends it scurrying into some dark recess.

A screen standing behind the bedhead, papered over that morning in a futile attempt to seal in the vermin it houses, is swarming with bed bugs. Flinging back the bedclothes, she catches them in the act and they flee across the mattress, tumbling over the edge, the theft of Lucy's blood evident in the red welts on her legs. She had seen these creatures before in some hospitals in England, but she had not been privy to their nightly feasts.

All she can do now is sit up in her chair with the wick fully raised, hoping the light will keep them away and wondering if her father had not been right in his disapproval of her chosen career, demonstrating his opposition by turning her portrait to the wall. How she looked forward to the accommodation promised in her contract: a comfortable furnished sitting room and bedroom suitable for a gentlewoman.

Tomorrow she will move to a clean, closely inspected room and will make sure her nurses are housed in a dormitory with four-poster beds, basins and mirrors while the Nightingale Wing is built.

The vermin had apparently not troubled Mrs Bethsheba Ghost, a predecessor to Miss Osburn. Titled Matron–Housekeeper, she had been in charge from 1852 to 1866. Bethsheba was a pardoned convict, worthy and conscientious, although known to fortify herself against these nightly invasions with a judicious serve of alcohol.

2
The Dumbstruck Patient

The Tutor School is housed on the first floor of the Nightingale Wing. The cheerful feeling I experience on first entering the sun-filled room is due to the resemblance to school rooms of my past. Two rows of school desks, exact replicas of the type I remember, are set out in the room. It is a comfortable feeling, being seated here on our second day, as I was happy at school, eager to learn and reluctant to leave.

Sister Breakall is seated at her desk, facing us, looking faultless, as does the made-up hospital bed behind her. The surrounding walls are decorated with various coloured charts of anatomical illustrations, and several trolleys are pushed up against the walls, stacked with metal objects large and small, all shining with a high brilliance. A life-sized doll is placed, rigidly expectant, in the sterile perfection of spotless and thoroughly ironed linen that makes up the bed. A white quilt is laid on top, strangely pinned around the end of the bed, with a large blue cross centred exactly where the patient's knees rest. Propped up on three pillows, the dummy seems to present an immobile, startled expression as though alarmed by this new batch of nine females coming to practise on her—all kinds of contortions forced on her limbs, bare body exposed, not to mention tubing of varying sizes pushed into unspeakable cavities.

We are told to sit at a desk and I slide into my chosen seat. Sister Breakall settles back in her chair, adjusts her starched cuffs and begins.

'Today we commence with the basic requirements for keeping the patient comfortable, as well as the presentation of an orderly ward.'

Her back is unbending and her posture seems to be a model for us to copy as we automatically push our buttocks towards the back rest and lift our shoulders: orderliness and deportment, numbers one and two of the 12 Indispensable Qualities Desirable in the Nurse listed at the beginning of the nursing notes placed on each desk.

'First chapter, please, in your *Modern Practical Nursing Procedures*.'

We dutifully respond, lift the thick, red-covered textbook and begin with Chapter I: 'How to Make a Bed'. One would think the making of a bed a simple task that would not need 16 pages of instruction, but there are 12 different types of made-up bed: the epileptic bed, the anaesthetic bed, the shock bed and one for an amputated leg are just a few. This will take a few days to work through and I am looking forward to getting down to something more cerebral—theoretical.

At this moment we must begin at the beginning: the 'plain' bed. Stripping, airing then remaking the bed, our plaster patient is sprawled awkwardly on a metal chair, arms and legs splayed and wide-eyed, as though viewing for the first time the starkness of the gangling skeleton hanging on the opposite wall. Perhaps we should give a name to our silenced patient but she will probably remain 'Dummy' just as our family cat always remained Kitty, for want of a better name.

I stand back admiring my handiwork. Linen and blanket corners squared perfectly, quilt flat and white as an ice floe, the centre cross an island of deeper ice blue; the overhanging pointed ends covering each front iron bed leg are lifted and folded in a square to each side and fixed with a plain pin. Pillows are vigorously plumped in their cases then stacked one on top of each other, openings facing away from the door. Working with the hands on a simple task can be strangely satisfying if the end result presents well, as it must for our Tutor Sister.

Immunisation was unknown in my infant days. This afternoon I experience my first injection, one of three painful doses administered at 10-day intervals to fulfil a course of typhoid immunisation. I wonder whether the typhoid bacillus still lurks in the aged hospital drains, putting staff at risk almost a century after typhoid cases were commonly nursed in the wards.

Rubbing my swollen deltoid muscle I marvel at modern science and the dead bacillus already working on stirring up my immune system.

Fever

Foul smelling—noxious vapours ... are thought to be the cause of the debilitating, life-threatening disease typhoid fever, common in Lucy Osburn's day and often referred to as colonial fever. A few weeks into their appointment in the colony, Lucy, Bessie Chant and new probationer Elizabeth Morrow are laid low with a high fever and abdominal pain. Head Surgeon Dr Alfred Roberts is called upon to assess their illness.

Lucy lies in a darkened room, the curtains pulled slightly back for his examination. Her flushed face is fiery below the cold compress covering her forehead, which does little to ease the blinding headache. Mary Barker, good practical nurse that she is, bustles in and out of the room, emptying the bucket of foul excrement and giving the best care to her superior. She is forced to dispose of the bucket's contents in the grounds at the rear of the Infirmary because toilets had not been installed during the building of the Main and South Wings. In addition, there are no taps, and so no running water, hot or cold. Buckets of water are carried to the wards from pumps in the yard, though they are mostly out of order. The irascible John Blackstone is known to deliberately complicate the situation by ordering the yardman not to man the pump when water is most needed. Ten years will pass before the Sydney water supply is connected to the Infirmary.

'Miss Osburn has the classic symptoms of typhoid fever,' Dr Roberts straightens himself at the bedside. 'Severe headache, high fever, diarrhoea.' Stepping back, concern is written all over his face. 'Her temperature must be rapidly reduced, you will be familiar with the treatment, Sister.'

Although Mary Barker is well versed in the application of the up-to-date, necessary procedures, she listens carefully. Dr Roberts is a man who insists on receiving the listener's complete attention, almost subservience, when giving his instructions.

'I will remove a volume of blood while I am here to help reduce the fever. The body is to be doused with cold water giving extra saturation to the severely inflamed skin areas.' He looks intently into the nurse's face: 'To be followed by cupping.'

He turns his head for further surveillance of Lucy's poor feverish body. 'And of course the scalp must be shaved.'

Eccentricity shows in the fashioning of his white beard, thick on the lower cheeks but not allowed to cover his chin. He strokes the flourishing moustache thoughtfully.

'Following your administration of these treatments I will have Miss Osburn moved to my house, quite close by, where she will have the greatest care given by my wife and her staff. I will carry out the leeching there.' This routine treatment is endured in the hope it will assist in a swift recovery; the repulsive creatures are sometimes inserted at the doctor's discretion into dark and private body channels through a glass 'leech tube', an essential aid carried in every doctor's surgical bag. Lifting his bushy eyebrows his nose sniffs the air, reminding Sister Mary of a bloodhound on the fox's trail. His eyebrows drop back into place, his forehead is forced down in a scowl.

'Ah, Sister, do you detect that foul smell, obviously rising from a leaking drain beneath the floor? Now we have the cause of Miss Osburn's illness, and more importantly the source. Miasma, as always, is the culprit!'

His medical bag is seized and smartly snapped shut.

Turned onto her stomach, her nightgown lowered to her waist, Sister Mary places across Lucy's upper torso the hot rims of heated cups, made especially for this purpose. The angry red circles indicate that the blood drawn to the surface will increase the circulation and alleviate the inner organs.

John Blackstone's distorted countenance appears like a nightmare in *her delirium, his devilish eyes burn into her back as she turns to run.*

The hefty scissors are efficient in Sister Mary's hands. Swathes of dark brown hair curl around the inner base of the basin. The snip-snipping around her ears is transposed to Lucy's brain as steel capped boots jarring on flagstones in Blackstone's pursuit of her.

Blackstone's recent appointment as Superintendent and General Manager in charge of male servants and male staff, before Miss Osburn's arrival, is a great surprise to Miss Osburn. She has expected to be in charge overall, and Blackstone lacks experience for the job. In many matters needing his co-operation he invariably opposes her requests, and as he threatens in her delirious state, he will be a nightmare to her in the years to come.

An intake of sustenance via both entries to the alimentary tract, with ice and soda water swallowed and nourishing enemas administered, Miss Osburn is nursed back to a reasonable state of health. She is determined to carry on and returns to work after three weeks. But her colleagues take longer to rally. Lucy suffers many bouts of illness during her Sydney career, always responding with a resilience that matches her strength of character.

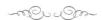

Following the evening meal we gather in our room, as it is the largest of the three occupied by our group. Sprawled out on our beds, we wait for the aspirin taken earlier to relieve our fever and soreness. One by one we drift off to the shabby share bathroom, seeking relief under a cool shower in a recess partitioned off from the next by a canvas curtain. Returning to the room we complete our summing up of the day. Pat, leafing through her copy of the three-page Code of Nursing Ethics, is holding in one hand a slim black Sobranie, the brand she constantly smokes, drawing in deeply between sentences. We are amazed at her daring, as smoking in bedrooms is forbidden. Seeing the alarm on her colleagues' faces she is unperturbed.

'Don't worry my loves, there won't be anyone snooping around at this time.' Surely the Home Sister will track down the awful stench from these black cigarettes, which must be fouling the air in the corridor outside. We continue to marvel at her determination to do things her way. We also feel slightly nervous that if caught out we will all get the blame.

A deep chuckle precedes her next sentence. 'I see that we must stand when speaking to those in authority.' She looks up in mock surprise with raised eyebrows: 'Do you think in our present lowly status we will ever be able to remain seated?'

Her eyes sparkle and, accompanied by a hearty laugh, she proceeds to act out the next piece of information. It is easy to see how her Drama School training has left its mark, making her the most extroverted in the group.

'A nurse should stand while speaking to a doctor, follow him and not precede; never be so bold as to become included in general conversation with a member of the medical staff.'

'I'm concerned about giving precedence to seniors at all times,' I comment and add, 'This involves every nurse and sister who is more senior and it includes passing through doorways. There are 51 sisters and 176 trainees, so we'll be lucky to make it through any doorway.'

'Including the dining room,' Judy, who has a healthy country appetite despite the quality of cuisine served at each meal, adds glumly.

We burst into laughter, ready to find fun at the smallest, silliest opportunity; conversation however flippant is merely a barrier against doubts over strict rules that we will, of course, adhere to. Pat continues marking the page with a forefinger while wagging the other.

'The etiquette of the army is to a certain degree repeated in the hospital.'

'Should we salute as we stand back at each doorway?' I ask with a giggle. Pat puts on a stern face reading out her findings like a magistrate lecturing on the law.

'Matron is held responsible for the conduct of each individual nurse,' adding thoughtfully, 'just as the captain of a ship has that responsibility. Sounds more like the navy to me.'

Prone to giving the occasional snort if surprised by something read, heard or seen, Pat carries on. 'Wait a moment, there may be someone serving in a lower role. According to this "maids are of a different class and social intimacy is forbidden".'

It could be that our place lies in the middle strata of social layers and we can neither converse with those above, that is the medical strata, nor those below in domestic service, almost positioning us on an elite level of our own.

Lights out, settling down I quickly drift into a sleep that is restless with nightmarish images. The patient silenced within her plaster body, who should be lying wrapped in the darkness of the Tutor School below, leaps out of her pristine bed and seeks me out with night eyes wider and wilder than those she wears by day. I run with the dummy hard on my heels, like a horseless Tam-O'-Shanter, down into the funnel of the spiral staircase, around and around, out through the doorway and into the open courtyard while my pursuer shouts, 'Wait! Do not pass through the doorway before me!' But I already have.

'You will be punished,' screams the dummy, and I wake, instantly swimming in a reactive sweat triggered by the typhoid vaccine and my nightmare.

3

The Wintry Sea

The Hotel Australia on Castlereagh Street is a splendid building both inside and out, especially the interior. There patrons meet moving across the gracious foyer towards one of the available bars, or sit allowing time to pass—the nonchalant newspaper readers, the relaxed observers or anxious ones waiting for the first sight of an advancing friend and others with pleased expressions when that friend arrives. Across the other side of the street stand two smaller hotels, The Carlton and Ushers. We choose Ushers for a celebratory pre-luncheon drink, marking the end of our first week and the whole weekend free to do as we please. This is how a hotel or club in London might look, or that is how I imagine.

We are indeed fortunate in having a workplace in such close proximity to pleasant meeting places and entertainment. A short walk two blocks down Martin Place and the choice is ours.

The group ascend the staircase to a higher floor and a quiet lounge, intimate within walls panelled in dark walnut. Comfortable heavy chairs, covered in a woven tapestry of muted autumn colours, are placed around glass-topped tables. The waiter is hovering at the edge of our circle: Pimm's No 1 is our choice. The mixture of Pimm's and ginger ale, with ice swimming on the top of the tall glass, is decorated with cucumber rind, orange slice and a cherry speared by a toothpick balancing on the rim. My first taste of this beverage is as rewarding as the presentation, but deceptive in its soft drink appearance. I settle back in the cosy, oversized chair. Soothing background sounds enter into the occasional quiet moments in our conversation: ice cracking in my glass, a woman's soft laughter from the far side of the room as her companion leans towards her, a tram bell clanging outside at the nearby intersection of Elizabeth Street and Martin Place.

I catch a glimpse of a young woman's reflection in the glass centre door panel on the opposite wall. Dressed in a grey tailored suit, if she were to stand a gathered peplum might be seen, forming the jacket's lower back below the waist. A cherry red cloche hat fits snugly on her head, almost hiding black hair that curls out around the edges.

Most women cannot resist observing their presentation in passing by a shop window or seated within range of a mirror and I am no different to the rest.

Let's not admit to vanity but call it a habit. I raise my glass in my pale grey-gloved hand feeling reasonably satisfied with my reflected image and more than satisfied to be sharing this hour with newfound friends.

I did not realise in that first week spent together that our friendship would be nurtured and grow and last for decades; or realise that this was a legacy of the previous 80 years, ever since the Nightingale Wing was built. Nurses, being required to live in, give support to each other through the tough times and form strong bonds.

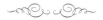

The city shuts down at lunchtime on Saturday and remains lethargic through Sunday: streets deserted, building doorways shuttered, department stores lifeless, cafe kitchens cold and milk bars silent, except for the passage of a few trams and an occasional tide of worshipers gushing out of the cathedrals, enveloping the pavement before rapidly drifting away towards their suburban roast dinners.

Most of the group are lucky enough to join families for the remainder of the weekend. Dulcie and Judy meet up with city relatives, and I am invited to stay overnight with Betty and Jack, my mother's friends whose semi-detached house sits on the craggy cliff facing the sparkling ocean rolling in onto Tamarama Beach. The sea, so close to the home I have left behind in Port Macquarie, where it is a five-minute walk and then a dive into the waiting surf, is a reminder to telephone my parents. Today the ocean is bracing on first entry then exhilarating as my body adjusts beyond the first plunge and later, wading out of the breaking surf, I find my laid out towel. Coconut oil slathered on arms and legs acts like a magnet drawing the sun down to broil the skin and bleach the fine fuzz of hair; a perfect solarium as I bask on the sand between the high tide water mark and the land's rocky edge. By the time I leave, my skin will be a rich rosy red, and once again I'll be hoping it will become the desired tan, which never happens. The need for relaxation in the summer sea requited, I board a tram and rattle back into the city's heart.

The third week in Tutor School is approaching, when each one of us will be allotted to a ward to work two evenings and one morning during the week. It's a taste of our true working environment and the real beginning of nursing training—more serious than the occasionally hilarious application and practice of bandaging each other or the 'dummy'. Every section of the human body can be expertly covered by one or more roller bandages, every cave where limbs and torso meet, limbs, appendages, torso and head, the method and pattern woven is described by name: reverse spiral, spica, fan, figure of eight. The real work of art is the capeline: two bandages are joined, one held in each hand, and worked around the head, one moving back and forward and the other horizontally, to invent a perfect cap.

The prospect of dealing with this initial ward experience may be daunting but I intend to tackle it in earnest.

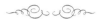

Pausing at the double doors of Ward 5, I grasp one of the long perpendicular handles, the brass grooved for an easier grip, pulling the door open. At 5.45 a.m. I step onto its bare boards. I draw in a deep breath. Then it is like diving headfirst into a wintry sea.

I remove my starched cuffs and place them on a shelf in the Nurses' Day Room, roll up my sleeves, automatically check to make sure my specially purchased surgical scissors and nurses' watch are tucked in respective pockets behind my apron. The scissors attached to a long piece of white tape secured by a safety pin, and the watch held by a chain. I calm my nervous state and the loud thumping in my chest by taking deep breaths as I move down the ward. A group of nurses stand around a desk in the ward's centre and the Night Nurse is reading out her report on the changeover to day staff.

I hover on the edge trying not to attract attention and listening to words that make little sense, hoping my expression shows some intelligence. At the end of the report, the Night Nurse drifts away towards the Day Room to remove the slippers worn to muffle her footsteps during her shift, then move onto breakfast and sleep. The Senior Nurse who is in charge until Sister comes on duty at 8.15 a.m. acknowledges my presence, gives me instructions as everyone else bustles away to carry out the routine each nurse is bound to do according to her year. How I envy their assurance in knowing exactly what their duties are.

The Code of Nursing Ethics must have made an impression, and surfaces at this point with a reminder 'that there is to be no familiarity with junior nurses' so I am sure no-one will pay me any attention. Therefore I am grateful to receive a wide and friendly smile from the other junior nurse on duty who is responsible for the right hand side of the ward as I am for the left.

Tea leaves saved from the oversized teapots and put aside the previous day have been rinsed, squeezed through a colander and placed on enamel plates. In unison the friendly junior and I pass down each side of the ward casting a handful of leaves under each bed, like biblical characters casting seed upon the ground. The purpose of this morning ritual is to settle the dust before sweeping commences, to help prevent airborne infection. I wield a straw broom behind the beds, which have been pulled away from the wall, fluff and dust suitably coated in tea leaves is swept out towards the ward centre, then pushed ahead of a wide soft broom by another nurse and the debris is collected in front of the ward doors.

During the registering of patients' temperatures, I move from bed to bed feeling more settled as the ward's layout and atmosphere become more familiar. Ward 5 is a men's medical ward situated on the second floor in the hospital's oldest section. It is also the top floor and faces out onto Macquarie Street. An open veranda runs the ward's length, empty except for a table where the patients' flowers are placed overnight, because it is not healthy to sleep and breathe in the same air as cut flowers. The plan of the large open wards in this original section of the hospital contain four service towers, one at each corner leading off the ward and used as pan room, treatment room and kitchen/day room, and the internal staircase fills the last. There are no lifts in these 1894 buildings. Patients needing to attend X-ray or similar departments are transported by chair or trolley to the nearest building containing a lift via a maze of adjoining bridges and loggias.

Early morning traffic is increasing now—a clattering of trays and cutlery emerges from the kitchen. The sun is creeping across the drawn blinds after washing the Domain with first light. The blinds that cover the tall windows are raised; someone turns off the lights; the correct number of windows is opened to a regimented height; and fanlights are adjusted. Foul air must be eliminated according to Sister Breakall, but we must also ensure there are no drafts, the ideal temperature is 68–70 degrees Fahrenheit (20–21 degrees Celsius).

Patients not obviously ill appear settled. Some are cheerful, speaking in raised voices and passing information to each other, a tip on the races or the quality of their night's sleep. Half a dozen others, seriously ill, are quietly enclosed within their present predicament; a few walking patients admitted for various tests move around chatting to those confined to bed.

An old man seated in the corner beside his bed must be feeling cold, wrapped as though it was mid-winter in his woollen Onkaparinga dressing gown. As I approach and place my tray of thermometers on his bed table, he is studying my face through his rheumy eyes, his mouth opening in readiness for me to slip the thermometer beneath his tongue.

'Why so serious, luv?' he asks as I shake the mercury down before placing the thermometer in the glass of disinfectant. 'You'll get used to it, you know.'

So, I think to myself, I must look as new as I feel and charting the temperature reading I feel the warmth, the flush of blood mounting my neck and colouring my cheeks. This coincides with movement at the ward entrance. The sudden thrust of an opening door and the resultant space is overwhelmed by the presence of a very tall woman.

Everyone capable of movement turns their attention in that direction.

She is dressed in a Sisters' uniform, not the blue commonly seen around the hospital and Nurses' Home, but a light grey. Her veil blossoms out stiffly on each side and is wrapped around her forehead low below her hairline, almost resting on her thick black eyebrows and piercing dark eyes. Her physique is angular with a hint of masculinity and it is obvious that on her early morning round as Deputy Matron she isn't going to overlook the slightest infringement of her strict expectations.

Sailing down the ward she checks right and left like a threatening man-o'-war in full sail, assessing the scene and the results achieved in the wake of sponging patients and bed making: tidiness must reign overall.

Height and corresponding level of blinds passes inspection; bedside lockers with books and magazines stacked on top shelf, slippers on bottom shelf, towel folded neatly behind with centre hospital name facing towards the door, pillow openings facing away from the door, beds an equal distance apart, quilts a uniform length. All in order until the man-o'-war sights a beacon glinting in the light of the entering sun: a lone methylated spirits bottle placed on a bed table has been overlooked at the completion of a patient's back rub.

Sister Bridgeman raises a hand, points a long admonishing finger at the offending article and her query is contained in a sentence that rises from the first overly stressed word and rumbles through to the last syllable.

'Who is responsible for leaving that bottle on that bed table?'

The junior nurse who had shown me a friendly smile is standing close by looking flustered and, following requirement No. 3 in Indispensable Qualities Desirable in a Nurse, Truthfulness, speaks out: 'Nurse Williams, Sister.'

This is a reference to a second-year nurse busily plumping up pillows nearby, her back to this scene, until called to remove the bottle. The look cast over the junior by the second year nurse must have felt like a covering blanket of hoary frost.

A sense of relief settles over the ward as with a surprisingly light turn on her strong legs the Deputy Matron changes course and moves towards the door. Immediately the Senior Nurse draws the glum-looking probationer, who has realised her act of betrayal, to one side.

'Nurse never on any account dob in a fellow nurse. Pretence is a good rule to follow.'

Truthfulness is therefore replaced by Indispensable Quality No. 4, Loyalty and doubt arises around No. 5, Accuracy.

Seven-thirty a.m. breakfast followed by a cigarette is a welcome break. My friends appear to have been allotted to second breakfast and I return to the ward at the same time as Sister Lileblad at 8.15 a.m.

Cuffs removed, sleeves rolled up I make myself known to her.

Seated at the desk checking the night report, there is no responsive expression on Sister's pretty face as she lifts her head to acknowledge my presence. She drops her remarkably blue eyes at once instructing me to get on with the routine already mapped out in Tutor School. In her cool, aloof way she continues to ignore me for the remainder of my shift, communicating any message through someone more senior.

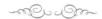

Indispensable Quality No. 6, Cleanliness, is a top priority, practised daily, in attention to self and in the care of patients and their environment. Just in case mothers of probationers have been slack in applying hygiene during their daughters' upbringing, a reminder in Tutor School notes lists 11 points on which to concentrate from daily bath through areas not to be overlooked, teeth, feet, daily bowel motion and non-participation in the taking of drugs and alcohol.

Cleanliness must be applied diligently to assist with the good health of others. Sister Breakall stresses how important it is to have a working knowledge of domestic affairs, hence the scrupulous ward cleaning. Microscopic bacteria lurk everywhere, on the skin, in the mouth, in the air or lying about ledges, or secreting themselves in crevices and on knobs, all of which need special attention.

Clean with firm, definite strokes, she instructs us and with my determination to tackle any task earnestly I begin at the ward entrance, partnered by a bucket of hot sudsy water and essential tin of Bon Ami. A line of painted medicine cupboards attached to the wall feels the pressure of a wrung out cloth wielded with my firm definite strokes. I have not progressed far before I feel a tap on my shoulder. Nurse Williams is standing behind me.

'Sister has sent me to say your efforts are painful to watch. Get a move on and for goodness sake leave some paint on the woodwork.'

So I move on to wipe lockers, bedheads, window ledges, overhead bed lights, metal chart backs and chairs until I reach the last bed without using the forbidden action along the way of flicking a dry duster, thereby polluting the air with the enemy—vengeful, invisible bacteria. Now I know why I have not glimpsed a domestic worker or cleaner anywhere. The State government convening in the adjacent north building must be delighted with the consequent cost saving in public hospitals due to the nurses' role as 'scrubbers', a term given to nineteenth-century hospital cleaners.

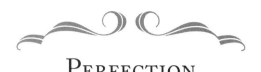

Perfection

Clean floors—clean air ... *clean everything, and when completed turn around and begin again. Learned from Florence Nightingale's sojourn in the British army hospital in Scutari, Turkey, cleanliness is a priority in the Nightingale method of nursing and essential in continuation of the patient's good health.*

An onerous task lies ahead in Sydney. The shabbily constructed building was erected by inexperienced builders who are more impressed with their winning the rum monopoly. Giving that acquisition first priority, they make a profit with an Infirmary raised on shallow foundations, over an inadequate drainage system and enclosed by rubble-filled walls creating a haven for vermin.

The open doorway to the female ward frames Miss Osburn's still figure. The silky rustle of her skirts sliding across bare boards is soft and her face shows concern on this, her first inspection following the Sisters' designated placements.

'Good morning Miss Osburn,' the quick movement of Sister Haldane Turiff towards her superior is immediately answered in Lucy's first impression.

'The first task for us Haldane, is to turn this miserable, chaotic scene into an orderly one.'

Admittedly it is too soon to have achieved any obvious advances.

A mishmash of ragged clothes, gowns, skirts and shawls are draped over bedheads and across window sills. Bags and rubbish are stuffed beneath the beds as though the room's interior had been designed and decorated by street urchins.

Haldane lifts her arm and sweeps her hand around to indicate the width and depth of the long ward.

'Being the colony's worst of the sick poor it seems they arrive with all they own, for fear of thieves stealing their goods away if they are left behind in their lodgings.'

'I will make it my business to obtain a bedside cupboard for each one,' Miss Osburn begins to move down the ward looking to left and right adding, 'as soon as possible. Then we can see to the washing and proper storing of their possessions.'

This will be a major suggestion to put before Blackstone, or possibly the Board, and one that may meet an automatic refusal. If so, perhaps Sir Henry Parkes will be her ally and speak up on Lucy's behalf. She has already gained ground in persuading Copeland Bennet, bath man and messenger, to help with the physical cleaning. When this is taken care of it will be time to conjure him into spraying and poisoning vermin. If too much opposition is met, Lucy is thinking of personally employing and paying a plasterer to seal up the worst cracks in the walls. A shudder runs through her body when the vision returns to mind, seen on a nightly round, of vermin crawling over a dying patient.

Her inspection brings her to the male ward. At the far end Sister Barker is standing looking up towards the pressed tin ceiling. It is difficult to tell from the doorway exactly why she is steadying a ladder and raising her voice as Miss Osburn hastens her steps down the space between the opposing rows of beds.

'Come down Nurse, at once,' Sister Mary Barker scolds. 'You may trip on your skirt and we'll be one nurse less.'

She is actually more concerned with impropriety than injury. The likelihood of the nurse displaying her ankles or worse, a length of leg, is most inappropriate. As it is, old Brannigan in the bed directly opposite is wide awake and making sure with one eye hidden that the other is peeping over the bedclothes. He is clutching a shortened ragged sheet from which pieces have been torn, for use as bandages or making poultices. A practice now strictly forbidden, it may have to be overlooked on occasion until the sheet supply is more plentiful.

Staring hopefully as the nurse hitches her skirt up in readiness for her descent, he is rewarded with a glimpse of a black laced-up boot and opaque black stocking. The thick leg covering, so important in Miss Osburn's mind, adds to the nurse's dignity and concealment of, that lustful word, flesh. The dense black stockings are secured with elastic garters that hollow out deep indentations in the mid-thigh.

'What is happening, Mary?' Miss Osburn asks Sister Barker, as the nurse arrives at the base of the ladder and her feet touch the ground. She is one of the more presentable and will be allowed to stay on. Three girls kept, the worst and altogether too dreadful will have to go. Three newly appointed Australian nurses will be engaged as trainees and, later, Miss Osburn plans to select more, a possible eight installed by July 1868.

'Nurse has taken it upon herself to attempt to brush the cobwebs off the ceiling,' and looking up Lucy sees that indeed there are filthy webs looped between corners like ancient fishing nets hung out to dry.

Sometimes selected mobile patients are encouraged to assist in menial tasks of cleaning, but the heavier work is part of the nurse's workload and in these early days, following more of Lucy's constant inspections, she is known to pick up a scrubbing brush and demonstrate how St Thomas's training has instilled the necessity of keeping walls well washed and window sills scrubbed. All cleaning is carried out during morning hours as Sydney's inadequate water supply is shut down by the city council between 3 p.m. and 6.30 p.m. each day.

'Many hands on the plough will reap a bountiful harvest and hard physical work is good for the soul,' is Miss Osburn's remark as she washes her hands, rolls down her sleeves and prepares to leave the ward. For good measure, 'Cleanliness is next to Godliness,' is an added afterthought.

Prayers are due to be said in the Chapel, and she must attend, setting an example by her punctuality.

In September 1868, the House Visitors on inspection of the great improvements achieved by Lucy Osburn and her nurses, give

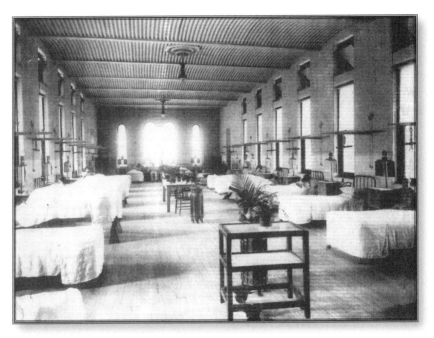

Male ward, Sydney Hospital circa 1890 (there had been minimal change by 1950). (Courtesy of Mitchell Library, State Library of NSW)

enthusiastic praise for the progress accomplished in such short time.

> *They manifestly have their heart and soul in the good work, and know how to go about this. Proofs are to be found in the scrupulous cleanliness of the wards and the absence of any offensive smell.*
> *(Hospital Visitor's Book, 13 September 1868, in Godden, page 149)*

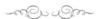

The Head Physician's twice-weekly round of his patients is due. The Senior Nurse hurriedly approaches before I can begin pouring the freshly squeezed juice, laboriously extracted by hand from a mountain of oranges. My sleeves are rolled down with cuffs in place as required when serving drinks. Her instructions are to leave this for the moment.

A more important task is given to me before the physician's arrival and I quickly wheel the trolley back to the kitchen area. I remove my cuffs and roll up my sleeves.

Move at a quick pace the Senior Nurse emphasised, and I begin to circle the ward, unplugging the bedside earphones, removing them from sight, stacked on the outer day room table in a pyramid of bakelite and wire cord. A source of irritability to the physician is distracting sound leaking from an unattended headphone. An occurrence once experienced was followed by his order for their removal before all future ward rounds.

The ward doors burst open, allowing entry to a varied entourage of medical associates. The close-packed group moves as one body but in order of importance and seniority. Head of the procession is the smartly suited Honorary Physician, wearing gold-rimmed glasses. A gold watch and chain is draped across the visible hint of a developing paunch.

The Registrar and Senior Resident in long white coats follow close on his heels. The Junior Resident in white drill jacket and pants, set off by a dark blue tie, is next. An almoner (social worker), dietician and a dozen or so medical students in short white coats are last through the doors, which swing shut behind them.

This prompts Sister to rise swiftly from behind the desk and move to greet the Physician who in turn acknowledges her with a cursory nod.

They gather each side of Mr Walker's bed. He is looking a little apprehensive at being the centre of attention for so many.

Having worked my way along the two opposing rows of beds, tidying, folding and smoothing the top sheet back over the straightened quilt of each one, Sister catches my eye and beckons. She whispers an order which sends me to silence the ward's solitary wardsmaid whose preparations in setting up for lunch clatter in the background. On re-entry to the ward I gently and slowly push the door open in case the hinges dare give out a squeak. Hovering near the pan room door I can observe the physician's manner, his imperious countenance creased at intervals by the set of a sardonic smile.

Light cast from a window adjacent to the bed, chancing on his glasses gives the gold rims a brighter gleam.

When confronted by his unapproachable personality, the Junior Resident, one of those responsible for the care of the Senior Doctor's patients, finds it difficult to explain or answer his questions. Perhaps the Physician's aloofness has been shaped by his genes and later intensified by five years' captivity as a prisoner of war. For the young doctor, a term trapped in the Physician's realm must be weathered and has no comparison with the punishments the older man must have suffered during his incarceration.

The students' answers to the Senior Doctor's questioning seem to satisfy him then, picking up the fluid balance chart from the bed table, he turns his attention to Sister, reprimanding her for the chart's incompletion. This is an important record in the patient's diagnosis and progress.

The Physician's body language barely alters, no raging or stamping of feet. A steely voice and cutting remarks are the weapons of intimidaton; an oversight not entirely her fault but, like the ship's master, she must carry responsibility for all areas.

I am relieved that the faulty chart isn't on my side of the ward. Feeling embarrassed for Sister I also forgive her for her earlier sarcastic reprimand over my meticulous cleaning of the medicine cupboards. I needn't have worried over Sister's hurt feelings. She always remains unflustered facing the physician with an inscrutable countenance, almost as pale as that of a geisha. Remaining silent, her bright blue eyes do not falter, levelling her gaze with his.

Mr Walker, centre of all the fuss, has an expression on his face that suggests this might be in some way his fault.

Removal of the Head Physician's presence signals re-insertion of earphone plugs into their wall sockets.

Visitors who had been hustled from the bedside out into the entrance foyer with the Physician's approach, are now allowed re-entry. Patients relax, stir in their beds and my carefully tidied top sheets are all askew.

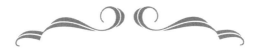

Dilemma

Tensions—tempers ... *lost, the use of violent language and abuse directed towards the nurses appalled Lucy Osburn.*

A long day and a typical one for Miss Osburn comprises many routine supervisory rounds throughout the Infirmary, beginning at 5.30 a.m. and continuing until late at night. Her energy has improved following her extreme illness and, feeling satisfied that the general cleaning of the wards is progressing well, she ascends the stairs with a more than usual lively step. Supper will be served soon and her appetite is quite sharp today.

As she approaches the entrance to the male ward a loud voice, full of hostility is clearly heard. She draws nearer and words become distinguishable as curses of an extremely violent nature.

'What is wrong now?' is her first thought. Quickening her pace, she arrives at the ward entrance.

A scene of anger and profanity, which might otherwise be comical due to the added action of a stamping foot by one of the involved persons, is blatantly directed towards one of her new trainees. The subdued girl seems overpowered by the verbal attack and Lucy is pleased to have appeared at just the right moment. The young doctor, his face ablaze, shows no embarrassment as the Lady Superintendent approaches. Her first thought is, 'Surely there is no wrong bad enough to be dealt with in this shameful manner.'

'Good morning, Doctor. Is there anything I can do to rectify this situation? You obviously feel wronged or perhaps disobeyed in some way?'

He has no reply, turning to walk away, his face seething.

'Go about your work, Nurse. Any grievances of medical staff must be

directed to the Sister-in-charge. Where is Sister Barker?'

Colour is gradually seeping back into the nurse's face, dispelling the wilted expression and she bustles down the ward seeking out Sister Barker.

Miss Osburn has witnessed several of these outbursts from junior medical staff. She thinks it cannot be a common occurrence, but obviously it is recurring. Without excusing these bad-mannered young men, perhaps this method of reprimand was used on the colonial nurses, in the belief it was the only approach possible towards that rag-tag lot. It will not do for the better style of young women replacing them. This situation must be resolved and quickly, or present trainees will not see out their training and staff shortages are the most difficult to rectify.

Miss Osburn's complaint is put before the hospital committee. She insists any grievances or complaints involving nursing staff be made to the ward's higher authority or to herself, rather than to the humble nurse. Miss Osburn adds that respectable women will not tolerate such insulting behaviour, pressing home the expectation that doctors will not vilify the Sisters or Miss Osburn.

This request is respected. The attitudes of junior doctors improve, but does not prevent the higher echelon of physicians and surgeons firing abuse at the Sisters.

Miss Osburn steps out with a confidence that grows, nurtured by her successes, but is occasionally forced to take one step backwards with any rebuff or criticism. She becomes bold enough to write to the Colonial Secretary on three occasions, making a formal complaint against the police, whose work, dealing with the city's worst, the homeless, incurable alcoholics, is similar to that of the nurses.

> *Sir, I wish to make this complaint an urgent one. There is no place in the Infirmary for the abusive, alcoholic patient, who with his dependence on this demon liquid or deprived of it, makes him a dangerous person to try and pacify in an overcrowded ward. The police are in*

the habit of depositing these disgraceful cases on our doorstep, too sick for prison but also totally unsuitable to be nursed in the Infirmary. I would urge you to look into this pressing dilemma.

Lucy re-reads her letter, folding it carefully in three with a sigh, then addresses the envelope. Copeland Bennett, the bath man and messenger, is called upon to deliver her correspondence to the Colonial Secretary's department a few streets away, in a newly built sandstone building of agreeable proportions. A reply is slow in arriving and contains a negative answer to a problem that will always be waiting for a solution.

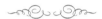

The friends get together for lunch at the end of the shift, discuss the morning's experiences and decide to avoid facing the evening meal in the dining room and at the same time breathe in different air as a brief respite.

Night is drawing in as we exit the hospital's rear gate and step out towards the Domain's soft green expanse, passing beneath the spreading canopy of a Moreton Bay fig tree. Twigs snap underfoot; a ruffled bird chortles in the leafy maze overhead; and a homeless hobo stretched out on a bench is startled and throws a curse in our direction, then turns to adjust his sheets of covering newspaper and regain warmth. A second vague figure shambles by in the gloom, moving towards another tree and bench to mark out his territory for the night. It is almost certain that at one time or another they have been deposited in Casualty by a police van, scrubbed by the wardsmen in Casualty's purpose-built bath, head and body hair dusted with DDT and released to rebuild a coating of filth.

Harry's Cafe de Wheels is parked in Woolloomooloo, a portable structure permanently placed where Harry serves his famous hot pies through the side counter of his caravan. The thick hardwood beam on the edge of a nearby finger wharf makes suitable seating. The venue is difficult to surpass, as brightly lit ferries slip by on an ink blue harbour. Trekking back through a black Domain under a moonless sky, we avoid the homeless, who in turn ignore us, a group of chattering females heading towards the scattered lights of a hospital bedding down for the night.

4

Social Intercourse

Each day I glance at the glass-enclosed noticeboard positioned on the left at the entrance to the Nurses' Sitting Room. Some oddments pinned to the felt look like they have been displayed there since the Nightingale Wing's inception. Not pausing to check on new additions, I am more interested in working carefully through the letterbox and the pigeonhole marked 'M'. One letter from home—I tuck it into my pocket to read quietly later in my room.

Janet and Barbara are seated in the row of chairs to the left of the phone booths and before I can seat myself Janet acknowledges me with a smile: 'Have you read the new notice on the board? Do go and have a look.'

Two third year nurses turning away from the noticeboard, obviously amused, make room so that I can check the recently positioned notice which reads:

> *It has come to my attention that there has been social intercourse between members of the medical staff and nursing staff. This practice must cease at once.*
> *Signed*
> *Matron Pidgeon*

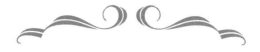

Relationships

Longing—love ... is sometimes thwarted, with a warning that such closeness is not suitable between two factions. A similar instruction might have been posted on a noticeboard in the newly completed Nightingale Wing by Lucy Osburn in late 1869.

At last the English Sisters are housed in a picturesque example of Victorian architecture, designed by Thomas Rowe in Gothic revival style. In her correspondence Miss Osburn has, pronounced the new wing 'very pretty'. The fine pattern of polychrome brickwork, rising up to form three floors with 38 rooms, has an aesthetic appeal and adds further grandeur to the main hospital precincts.

The Sisters are delighted with the single-room accommodation given to each one and they feel their status in the colony must be emphasised, now they are quartered in a building that has the unusual distinction of being especially designed to house nursing staff. Other colonial and British hospitals provide shared rooms for the nurses, adjacent to the wards, and the Sisters are often given single accommodation fashioned out of any available nook or cranny.

Sister Annie Miller bustles into her room, which is delightfully redolent of new furniture, bed-linen and curtains, described by a contemporary as being 'beautiful ... furnished and fitted up better than most nurses could hope for'.

She carries a parcel under one arm and a bunch of flowers in her hand, both purchased in the town. A vase is unwrapped, filled with water from the nearby jug and the flowers carefully arranged. It is not often Annie spends money on impractical purchases, but these have been bought for a special reason. She moves to dispel the smell of fresh paint by opening one of the windows overlooking the green Domain.

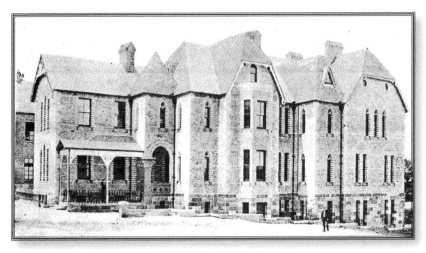

The original Nightingale Wing, completed in 1869. (J.F. Watson, The History of Sydney Hospital 1811–1911, Government Printer, 1911. Courtesy of Sydney Hospital Medical Library)

The view carries on down over the treetops and onto the bright blue harbour.

She pauses to admire herself in the oval, full-length mirror, suspended on a frame and glinting in the light from the open window. One of these has been placed in each room, an essential accessory in any woman's bedroom. John Algar, member of the Hospital House Visitors' committee, on a tour of inspection of the new wing, is responsible for their thoughtful addition. He also makes a comment on the beds appearing comfortless. But not to Annie Miller, whose happy frame of mind sees all things as being satisfactory.

She takes note that her choice of daisies enlivens her environment. The yellow blobs of colour, centred in wheels of white petals, diffuse an earthy scent of foliage. She refuses to think of the extra years she has not confessed to in her application to join the Australian expedition, stating her age as 34. Her Sydney colleagues assume she is some 10 years younger.

As promised, when the clock strikes 7 p.m. there is a light tap on the door. Nervously Annie moves across the room and, as expected, the portly figure of Dr Rudolf Schuette, Resident House Physician, fills the open doorway. Despite his 56 years, the fluffy beard taking over a good part of his features reveals very few grey streaks. His thick hair, refusing to lie flat in combed neatness, covers his head in a state of unruliness. Annie in her continuing blissful frame of mind sees the image of an exceedingly attractive male.

'Good evening Annie.' Dr Schuette steps across the threshold, while she extends her hand towards one of two deep armchairs.

'Excuse me for a moment and I will arrange for a tea tray to be sent up.' Annie's cheeks are flushed with pleasure at the thought of being able to cater for his needs and, more importantly, that he has come to visit at his suggestion.

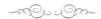

'We have many things in common, Annie. Subjects of interest which we can compare.'

The evening progresses as they discuss his degree obtained in a German hospital, while she exaggerates aspects of her training at St Thomas's before arriving in the colony. The conversation is sweetened by the sipping of tea and the very likely prospect of future tete-a-tetes.

The only conflicting opinion arises during the evening from his disapproval, indeed he accentuates the immorality, of women nursing men and she in her most genial way, opposing his view.

'The Nightingale system is insistent on this,' Annie explains, 'and Miss Osburn will soon implement this in its entirety.' Enlarging on her point she continues. 'This change has to be accepted and will be, because of the reverence bestowed on Miss Nightingale and her nurses in the light of their devoted nursing of soldiers during the Crimean War.'

These meetings with Dr Schuette continue for the rest of the week, from 7 p.m. to 9 p.m. His visits becoming a regular occurrence over many weeks.

Sister Annie returns from another visit to the town and this time the parcel carried under her arm is opened to reveal a pair of best-quality men's slippers made up from rich, red velvet, purchased in the markets. The shipment from England is newly arrived that morning. She cannot wait to thread her embroidery needle with the gold thread, also purchased that morning, and begin to stitch a decorative pattern across the insteps. The following week sets the seal on a routine that ensures his outfitting is perfected by freshly laundered shirts and collars.

'My dear, you are too good to me.' Dr Schuette steps through the doorway, his anticipation fulfilled as he quickly surveys the room.

As expected, tended to by her own hands, his pristine shirts hang on the wardrobe knob in readiness for collection.

Haldane Turriff is so incensed with Annie's behaviour, she is forced to ferociously stride the length of corridor to Miss Osburn's office. Barely pausing to knock she enters the room. Reporting deficiencies in other people's behaviour always sets off an exciting thrill through her body and here it comes once more as she halts with a stomp in front of the Lady Superintendent's custom-made desk.

'I must bring to your attention, Miss Osburn, something I have just witnessed. Sister Miller has gone out of her way to chase after Dr Schuette in a hospital corridor. Then she detained him, standing very close to his body, looking into his eyes while playing with his guard chain!' Haldane draws in a deep breath, the thrill stirred up by this report is fading so she must fan it to restart the flame.

'She takes every opportunity to pursue him. I see it happening regularly and therefore interferes with her concentration on the true purpose in being here.'

Sighing, Lucy slowly puts down her pen and lifts her eyes, looking into Haldane's cross face.

'I will give this problem attention Haldane. A notice, briefly worded but to the point, will be placed in the Sisters' sitting room and I will move her to the surgical ward so that she will not have contact with him.'

Haldane, as always, has the last word. 'Dr Schuette is a vulgar man.

His visits into our domain should not be tolerated.'

Very soon the situation rectifies itself.

Dr Schuette's absence for one whole week sends Annie's mood into a gloomy downward spiral.

Sister Turriff strides the corridor once more, lifts her skirts and moving upwards takes the length of the cedar staircase with great skill and swiftness. One could not have hoped for news more thrilling than this to pass on. She bursts into Annie's room and blurts out her message.

'Dr Schuette has taken time off in order to marry.'

Poor Annie, with a sensitivity stronger than most, feels the blood draining from her face and whispers, 'It can't be true. I don't believe it.'

'It is all over the hospital. I have said all along he is a vulgar man.'

How cruel life can be. Like a bitter medicine such a blow can be difficult to swallow and in this case presents side effects for Miss Osburn to correct. Annie's sorrow turns into hysterics, needing to be placated with three weeks' bed-rest. Treats are offered to lift her spirits: tidbits bought at the markets, ale when needed and red wine for supper to help induce sleep. Everyone knows of the rejection, the most difficult hurt of all to bear.

The real cure is achieved with Dr Schuette's return to visiting the room at the top of the staircase in the Nurses' Wing, although he is a married man. His visits are undisputed with his assurance that Annie Miller, now diagnosed with an abdominal aneurism, is his patient.

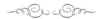

Lucy Osburn experiences her own grief over lost love.

That emotion is introduced with the purchase of a black and tan terrier. His affection knows no bounds and neither does his enthusiasm with his effusive greetings. When he sees Lucy, his small legs are triggered and his body reacts like the repeated bouncing of a rubber ball. Licking Lucy's face with his pink tongue, the warmth in hugging another live being swells in her chest like true love. Catching the rats that abound around the Infirmary is his special expertise. No rodent dares enter the Nightingale Wing while he grows into maturity, until Lucy receives a House Committee request to banish him from the Infirmary.

Lucy's loneliness is paramount with the little terrier gone and the rats move in once more.

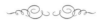

Eighty years later, in 1949, no male would dare set foot beyond the Visitor's Sitting Room, but despite Matron Pidgeon's concerns about fraternisation, a high percentage of doctors and nurses marry, thrown together during long working hours, and with little time to socialise outside the hospital.

I have other ideas and preferences—the often improbable daydreaming of a young girl spurred on by a passion for the unrealistic world of movies. Janet and I share that same passion.

A new movie is showing at the Embassy Theatre in Castlereagh Street. *I Know Where I'm Going* stars Roger Livesey in the lead role, a Scottish laird in a story set on a remote Outer Hebridean isle. Filmed in black and white, the setting of his ancestral home within a mist-shrouded castle adds to the romantic atmosphere. An unexpected stranding and emergence from the foggy night is played out by the heroine, Wendy Hillier.

Re-entering the real world, crossing the street and passing by David Jones into Elizabeth Street, I remark that Roger Livesey's build is well suited to the kilt. We step up and seat ourselves in the compartment aboard a toast-rack tram, heading out to Bronte and Janet's parents, who have invited me to stay Saturday night at their home, the top half of a duplex overlooking the sea.

Riding the tram, swaying up Oxford Street, the movie's theme tune is persistently running through my head. Outside, balancing deftly and swinging hand over hand to the call 'fares please', the conductor grips the handles above the tram's side walkway. Pushing

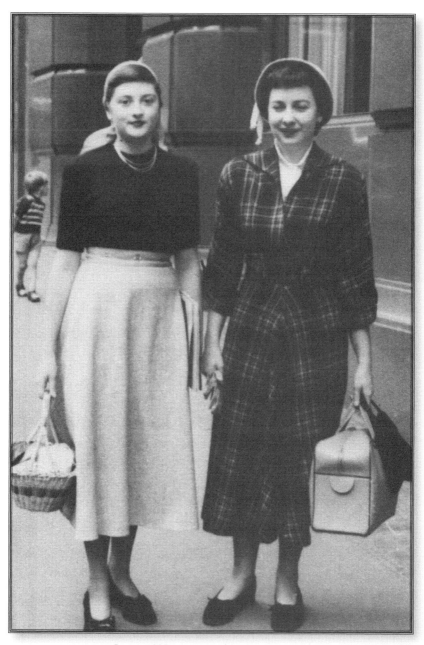
Janet and Norma, 1949. (Author photograph)

the tickets into my purse I share my thoughts with Janet.

'I think I'll marry a Scotsman. I am of Scottish descent and empathise with all things Scottish.'

'You are an incurable romantic and still under the spell of that film,' she replies and adds a question I can't answer.

'Where will you find this Scot and do you expect real estate, too? A castle perhaps with two huge deerhounds as well, like the two always sniffing at the hero's heels?'

The stone gates of Centennial Park leading into the wide acreage of lush parkland appear on the right then quickly fall behind. We rock in the soothing rhythm set by the tram's speed. After a short silence and, not wishing to quash my hopes, Janet in her kind way adds: 'I'm a romantic too. A lively imagination and a few hopeful dreams do no harm and considering we work in a scenario sometimes agonisingly realistic why not have a few unlikely dreams?'

She had been distressed during that week by the first death she had witnessed, that of a young, married 26-year-old man, diagnosed with leukaemia. She had said little about that. I had yet to deal with seeing this ending of a life, which is inevitable, unlike my wish to meet a stereotype fashioned in my mind after seeing a movie.

Ahead the ocean expanse at Bondi sparkles, framed in shops left and right, clear blue sky above, the road ahead dipping towards the sea and out of the picture. The conversation moves on to other desires to suit the body's needs as the tram swings to the right following the tramway to Bronte and we speculate on what Janet's mother may be cooking for dinner.

Janet's parents prove to be welcoming and make delightful company. Her mother has a keen sense of humour while her father, with his shock of wavy grey hair, reveals the kind disposition and brown eyes passed on to his daughter. And the meal served surpasses our expectations. Juicy breadcrumbed cutlets are served from a centre platter, on either side steam vapour rises with the lifting of lids from vegetable dishes. Home-made ice-cream follows, speared with an Arnott's wafer biscuit accompanied by whole baked Granny Smith apples stuffed with sultanas and cinnamon.

Following dinner we help clear the dishes while Mr Burstal retires to the lounge room to listen to the seven o'clock news. Drawing on his pipe and creating a hovering smoke screen over his special corner, he is seated beside the radio console concentrating on the newsreader's polished British accent. My father is probably doing the same at that moment, tuned into the country reception so often sparked with static. The pungent scent of burning pipe tobacco is a manly aroma and taken for granted, but before I light an after-dinner cigarette I ask for permission, which is readily granted.

Flicking through a stack of sheet music kept in the piano stool Janet unearths the composition she hopes will be found near the bottom of the ageing pile. Turning off the radio Mr Burstal leans back into his armchair and proudly looks on as Janet places the music sheet on the open piano lid and her mother, seated at the keyboard, loosens her fingers, running them over the keys before commencing the introduction to the song.

Janet's voice lifts the black notes off the page, combining them through her rich, deep, lower tones, sweet and strong in the higher, making the room vibrate. With six years of piano study behind me, my ingrained love of music appreciates, indeed is astonished by Janet's rendition of the traditional folk song featured in our afternoon movie.

> I know where I'm going
> And I know who's going with me
> I know who I love
> But the dear knows who I'll marry.

I have stockings of silk
Shoes of fine green leather
Combs to buckle my hair
And a ring for every finger.

Some say he's black*
But I say he's bonny
The fairest of them all,
My handsome, winsome Johnnie.

Feather beds are soft
And painted rooms are bonny
But I would leave them all
To go with my love Johnnie.

I know where I'm goin'
And I know who's going with me
I know who I love
But the dear knows who I'll marry.

* *Ugly*

Driving us back to the hospital the following afternoon, Mr Burstal approaches Macquarie Street via the road climbing the rise from Woolloomooloo. Passing the Domain on the left, cricketers in their crisp creams are spaced out across the rich open green reserve, the afternoon shadow of Victorian-styled Sydney Hospital lengthening across the scene. Mr Burstal lifts a hand from the steering wheel and gestures towards the players. He speaks with a break in his voice and reveals the true Anglophile within: 'There'll always be an England.' And I, secretly amused, think of my own father who would never voice such a sentiment, despite his mother having been born in Lincolnshire. For him there is no place on earth as great as his birthplace and his father's, in country New South Wales.

Stepping out of the car and facing the heavy stone buildings, the grand stairs leading up to the Administration Building, my heart sinks. Each time I return to the hospital following a day off, this is my reaction and I wonder if this feeling of doom will eventually dissipate.

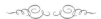

Daybreak. Ward 5 is stirring; the impetus quickens; patients wake; sound increases; ward traffic multiplies; the open ward is busy with planned activity. My task is to put in practice a procedure demonstrated during the week in Tutor School and carried out on our lifeless patient of neuter gender: a full sponge bath on a completely helpless bed patient.

Watching my patient with apprehension and the struggle this middle-aged man is having, propped up on three pillows, gasping behind the rubber oxygen mask to fill his air-starved lungs, compassion is my utmost emotion. His acknowledgment of my presence is shown by the intermittent raising of his eyelids accompanied by a fluidy groan.

Mr Jackson is not an old man. The age written on his chart is 55, but his illness has prematurely aged him, sallowed his skin, greyed his hair and depleted his muscles. His failing heart throbs visibly and erratically in his neck. Theoretically I should lay him flat, but he is too breathless. Removing one pillow I ease him down gently and decide swiftness while being thorough will achieve the best result for both of us. Areas are exposed and sponged in a definite order with as little laid bare as possible. It is important to respect the patient's dignity, oblivious though he may be to his present vulnerability. This constant reminder expressed by Sister Breakall is impressed into my brain. A towel placed under each part uncovered, head, neck, ears then arms, chest, abdomen, hips lathered, dried (not forgetting care of the

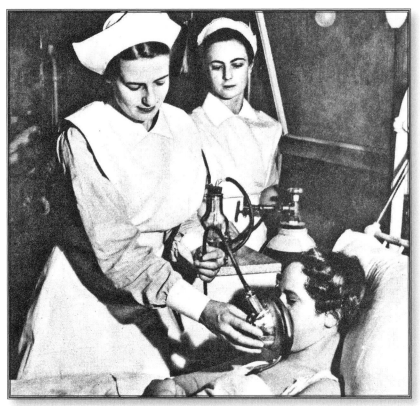

A senior nurse supervises a probationer in the administration of oxygen, circa 1940. (Pix magazine, courtesy of Mitchell Library, State Library of NSW)

umbilicus), Mr Jackson to all appearances is unaware of my care. Occasionally breathing out then not breathing in as rapidly as I would wish spurs me on. Careful observation, perhaps the most desirable trait in the efficient nurse is top of my list as I hold my breath until he inhales his next.

My care of Mr Jackson's hygiene arrives at the genital area, my first sighting of the private male area, previously studied only as a diagram in *Sears Anatomy and Physiology*. The sketch is obviously based on a much larger scale in comparison with this appendage finally located, dealt with swiftly, as per my original plan, but without the thoroughness Sister Breakall would expect.

The water must be changed before tackling thighs, calves, feet, while some difficulty is experienced with the immersion of each foot in the bowl placed on a towel at the end of the mattress. Lastly the back is sponged and flesh rubbed with methylated spirits, dusted with talc powder, and the bed linen changed with assistance. His supply of oxygen is checked on the gauge attached to a tall black oxygen cylinder next to his bed. Not knowing if he can feel my fingers wrapped around his hand I give a gentle squeeze.

I hope this gesture reassures him that the lifting of limbs, removal of clothes and the rolling about, all the movement which must be stressful for him, is over for now.

Propped up once more, my patient is re-clothed in fresh pyjamas and immaculate bed linen and I experience a feeling of achievement. The bed screen supported on a heavy metal frame is removed by folding in each side across the end section. This hugely cumbersome affair on wheels is trundled back to centre ward, having a mind of its own, all the way resisting any direction I push or pull it in. All accessories are stowed away, including the meths bottle, just as Sister Bridgeman pushes the ward door open and, despite his sad condition, Mr Jackson presents as pretty much shipshape.

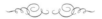

The social side of life remains uncomplicated but pleasant, centred around my nursing friends, my only male contact being attending to male patients and the fathers of my friends. An invitation to spend the night with a friend's family is a saving grace whenever days off coincide.

A street photographer always waits on the same Martin Place corner and snaps us in various pairs as we make our way to the tram stop or railway station.

Walking briskly down Martin Place towards Wynyard our

destination would be Barbara's home in Ashfield. Imaginable worries and work constraints left behind, our black and white images are captured for posterity by his camera.

We reach Pat's home by tram—she lives with her grandmother due to some upheaval in her parents' life. The house is one of many constructed in the style of a Californian bungalow situated next door to a racing stable in Kensington. The soft neighing, a hoof stamping, the equine snort and head shaking peculiar to that animal drifts into the darkened bedroom as we lie on the edge of sleeping. It's a comforting and homesick-producing sound to a country girl, although I had not experienced being seated astride a horse—our family live in the town. Further on, the tramline reaches another bungalow close to the sea at Maroubra: another place of respite, spent with June's family, with the added joy of sea swimming and home cooking. What a blessing to have these diversions from institutional living.

At the end of the morning shift the hospital dining room is avoided if possible. The tradition of eating, or rather bolting down in case of being caught, leftover servings of untouched patients' lunch while hiding behind the Day Room door is quickly seized upon by new trainees. This fare is a minimal improvement and eating here adds time to the off-duty afternoon hours. It also deprives the piggery's inhabitants when the special waste bucket designed to hold leftover scraps is collected by the 'pig man'. I doubt whether the Sisters eat behind the Day Room door, as this would be setting a bad example and I wonder if they are rewarded with better meals, having survived training and been elevated to a higher sphere.

Social Graces

Fraternisation—Intermingling... *are lacking in the Nightingale nurses' lives, with few or no diversions from the heavy load of hard work. The enjoyment of eating is one of life's few pleasurable pastimes open to them and hospital food must fill the greater part of this necessity. For the principal meal at 2.30 p.m., meat was served with vegetables and a sauce, followed with a pudding, often a fruit pie. At 5.30, tea was taken, and later the nurses sat down for a light supper of cold meats, eggs, cheese, bread and butter.*

In her writings to Miss Wardroper at St Thomas's, Miss Osburn describes their diet as:

> Toast, butter without limit, chops and beef steak daily—luncheon, unlimited cheese, butter and claret wine (no beer being drunk in the country).
>
> (Godden, page 159)

She closes her communication on the Sydney fare, describing the food as being served with noteworthy accoutrements, fit for ladies of a gentle persuasion and matching their newly completed establishment. These are silver-plated cutlery, cut glass tumblers and damask table linen.

The description of their daily diet is viewed differently by Sisters Miller and Chant, who complain to Lucy Osburn that they are 'starved', despite the variety of foods served, while Lucy regards their complaints as another example of their habitual grumbling. Seated in the Sisters' Dining Room, she is embarrassed when the colonial Sisters, better educated and better mannered than their British counterparts, have to eat at the same table, especially with Eliza Blundell and her poor manners.

The Nightingales have no opportunities to learn from observation of other peoples' table manners while eating in private homes. In these early months a social life is non-existent: their lives are shared with each other in the Nightingale Wing or with colonial staff on duty, attending patients or praying with other worshippers in chapel or at church. They are bored and discontented, and avoid shopping because goods in the colony are expensive. The town is dull after London.

So resentment grows for Miss Osburn's 'finding refinement' in the colony, as she herself explains it, cultivating growing friendships with prestigious people in high places, such as Captain Arthur and Elizabeth Onslow of Camden Park, where she finds respite from her difficult duties. Three weeks' leave in the summer heat of February is spent at Camden Park and some time at Throsby Park, summer residence of the Belmores at Mittagong. She admits to the joy brought about by her inclusion in visits to such refined houses.

The effervescent governor's wife, Lady Belmore, and the commodore's wife, Helen Lambert, are ladies who visit the Infirmary regularly to read to the patients. Lady Belmore is particularly kind to Lucy, sending a carriage to take her to Government House or calling in with an invitation to take a drive into the country—a favourite excursion is to the lighthouse at South Head.

The nurses are not invited to any of these places, nor anywhere else. Circulation with the local population is placed further out of reach by their criticism of the town's citizens and their forebears, 'all mixed in with convict blood'.

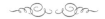

But Bessie Chant falls in love with a patient while in charge of the accident ward.

A personable young man is admitted and diagnosed with a dislocated hip: his injury is extremely painful. Standing beside his bed *and gazing down on his contorted face, cleanshaven clear skin, thick black hair splayed across the pillow, teeth clenched then relaxing as the sedation sets in, a row of straight white teeth are revealed as he smiles up at her. For Bessie, a 30-year-old Anglican widow, the stirrings of sexual attraction are heightened, not just for the desirability of his good looks, but because she is also intrigued by his eligibility and apparent respectability. Despite learning his occupation is that of a railway stoker he has obviously had a good upbringing.*

Yes, undoubtedly a cut above the many lesser citizens of Sydney's population that she attends every day.

The Surgeon and his assistant move away from the bed into a corner out of earshot and after a few minutes of serious discussion, accompanied by whisker stroking and eyes cast to the floor in concentration, as though surveying the floor's state of cleanliness, they return to the 'dislocated hip's' bedside. Bessie hovers anxiously nearby and is devastated to learn that her patient is to be transferred to Melbourne for specialist treatment. There are complications unable to be treated at the Infirmary.

The special week of giving her patient devoted attention is coming to an end. She abruptly turns away, hurrying to seek privacy in the adjoining linen room. Alone in the dim, dark space she lays down her head, nestling her nose into the fresh odour of newly washed linen and sheds bitter tears.

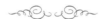

A light knock on Miss Osburn's office door and permission given to enter, reveals Haldane Turiff with a letter clutched firmly in one hand. In her eagerness to present her find, her shoe catches on the rug, but swiftly regaining her balance, she hands the letter to her superior.

The letter stems from Haldane's daily ritual, examining the Sisters' mail while unseen, for one never knows what can be assessed from postmarks or the sender's address. Haldane is positive she will be rewarded one day with some evidence that proves another Sister is guilty of a misdemeanour.

This letter, lying on the large blotting paper pad, has a Melbourne postmark. It is addressed to Sister Bessie Chant.

Haldane's expression is one of triumph and she leans forward eagerly. 'Perhaps you should censor this communication, Miss Osburn.'

Credit must be given to Lucy for hesitating and scowling at her Sister, but her indecision passes and curiosity wins the day. Haldane places emphasis on her suggestion in order to move things along.

'I have personally seen Sister Bessie hanging over this man's bed and I am ashamed to say, kissing him. Although the young man pleaded with her to desist she would not. Sister Bessie's sexual adventures have been very prominent.'

Miss Osburn's eyebrows lift and her jaw drops. Haldane seizes her next opportunity. 'Sister Chant is easily swayed by attention from the opposite sex and this should be monitored before she becomes too involved and our profession is discredited.'

Her eyes narrow as Lucy lifts the letter opener.

'Yes, you are right. I have enough opposition as it is and a scandal is just what my opponents will delight in.'

She makes a quick slit in the envelope. Skimming through the contents, she clasps the letter against her chest.

'It's a love letter from the "dislocated hip". He is coming to Sydney to claim her!' *Beneath her voile headpiece Lucy feels the cold perspiration breaking out over her scalp.* 'I will answer this letter personally, telling him to cease this correspondence or he will be reported to the Colonial Secretary. No more love in the accident ward, or any other department. Please wake Sister Bessie and tell her to report to me at once.'

Aroused from her sleep following a night on duty, pulling on her petticoats and uniform, Bessie descends the stairs rubbing the sleep from her eyes.

Poor Bessie, not fully awake and vulnerable, sways before Miss Osburn. She appears penitent when faced with her 'sexual adventure' and promises to cease communication with her would-be lover.

As always, Miss Nightingale is kept informed by Miss Osburn. Answering from her chosen confinement in her London bedroom, the older woman rebukes Lucy for opening another's personal letter. As the time-frame is eight months for a letter to reach England and the answer received on return, that chapter in Bessie's life has faded into the background and is replaced by another more complicated matter, eleven months after the accident ward affair.

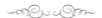

One patient is naked from the waist down, standing at the bedside and rifling through his neighbour's locker in search of pyjama pants. The garment located, he steps quickly into the legs and drags them up over his skinny flanks, assuring his fellow invalid they are only being borrowed. He is anxious to join the other patients gathered around a narrow window, jostling for enough room to spread elbows across the window sill and ogle Sister Bessie Chant. Well advanced in pregnancy Bessie is passing across the courtyard and if she hears the taunts from above she shows no recognition. Bessie's condition is fuel for the sniggering gossips in the small village-sized institution, where the news is spread as fast as fire can consume a small settlement.

The gathering around the window in their mismatched attire are shooed back to their beds with Sister Barker's arrival. She will be sure to inform Lucy Osburn of this scene, during her tea break.

Lucy in turn, writing to Florence Nightingale with her lengthy descriptive versions of gossipy happenings in Sydney, describes in detail Bessie's lapse, while adding complaints about the tempers and moods of the others. She neglects to concentrate on their hard work and nursing abilities, just as the records in her Nurses' Register tend to add more about their personalities and private lives than their well-intentioned efforts.

As for the Bessie Chant episode, here is another disgrace to the wearing of the nurse's uniform, into which Bessie now barely fits.

Early one morning in November 1869, without confiding in

anyone, Bessie quietly leaves the Nightingale Wing and slips out into Macquarie Street. Later in the day she is secretly married to William Simpson. [Author's note: unfortunately we do not know if this is the 'dislocated hip'.] She then resigns from the Infirmary.

Perhaps feeling remorse at her invasive actions over Bessie's letter, Lucy is instrumental in gaining a secure position for William as a stationmaster in the Blue Mountains. In return Bessie and William name their second child Lucy Osbourne Simpson, spelling the name incorrectly, as so many people do.

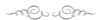

My teens are catapulting by, with a nineteenth birthday fast approaching and, when I listen to my friends' discussions, relationships are an important subject, but the opportunities for meeting someone of the opposite sex are scant.

Social interaction between nurse and patient does not get a mention in the Code of Nursing Ethics. Intimacy in this relationship is in a different category, although physical closeness is real. Some nurses do marry patients. With such brief experience, I find sexual attraction unimaginable in the day-to-day occupation of nursing and, until this point, the pace required to get the job done leaves only fleeting moments of light conversation with patients. The paramount emotion when dealing with the sick is compassion. These are my thoughts two months into nursing, when I am nearing the completion of Tutor School and very much a neophyte.

5
Inner-city Life

Results posted on the noticeboard show that no-one has failed the end of Tutor School examination, and we are assigned to full-time ward rosters.

Always poor by the arrival of the next payday, wages are collected from Matron's office in cash sealed in a small brown envelope. The amount is also small—less than £2 after deductions for board and lodging. A lot of juggling will be necessary to cover all the places and entertainment, so close to hand, that I like to frequent.

Living in Macquarie Street in the city's centre is one of the great advantages about training at Sydney Hospital, with the convenience and availability of things to do when off duty. Go out through the front gate, turn left, pass the gentle Georgian architecture of St James' Church and the northern end of Hyde Park, and David Jones department store is a short step away. Racks of the latest fashion pieces to flip through; tea and scones to enjoy in the seventh floor cafeteria; then riding the wooden-stepped escalators back down and emerging through the high vaulted ceiling into the spacious ground floor where the air is spiced with French perfume. An alternative ride is in the speedier lifts that are attended by a uniformed employee reciting the list of goods stocked on each floor as the door slides open. There are many other special emporiums to browse through, their floors filled with wonderful goods.

The post-war period has passed. Clothing rationing is a thing of the past and we are on the threshold of the 1950s. Nearby are Farmers, Hordern Brothers, Mark Foys and Curzons. With its modern interior, Curzons is impressive, finished with glass and chrome fittings, though the marble is perhaps not authentic.

The ground floor of Curzons is supervised by the floorwalker, Mr Hocking. Well known to me now, I had encountered Mr Hocking when, early that year, I had spent six months serving lady customers: his dark pinstripe suit and red bow tie are flawless; his fine profile, youthful skin and hair slightly flecked with grey and never a strand out of place is worn slightly longer than is usual; short back and sides, the common cut for men, would never have been the instruction given to his barber. I had worked on the glove counter, where the ritual began with insertion of a glove stretcher to loosen the glove's leather fingers, followed by dusting in a film of talc powder before slipping the glove onto the customer's hand as she rested her elbow in a specially moulded rest.

That hopeful trial of city life was shared with my friend from schooldays, Kay, who worked on the third floor, which was wholly devoted to the busy hat department. Boarding in the draughty spare back room of an Enfield house, bathing in water heated by a recalcitrant chip heater that stomped and puffed angrily beside the bath, did not last. We happily returned to the country with sore feet and aching backs to rethink our careers.

My next career move would continue to produce an aching back and feet, but Macquarie Street offers much better access than Enfield to the plentiful movie houses, Art Deco dream palaces: the State, Regent, Plaza and Prince Edward theatres are top of the list.

Hat and gloves, essential daywear accessories, are removed as the lights dim. I stand in unison with the other patrons for the national anthem, 'God Save the King', then settle into the velvet seat as the latest Cinesound newsreel begins, a misty black and white showing of the latest catastrophes, ending with a short, humorous segment of local interest.

The discovery of the Savoy Theatre in Bligh Street where subtitled continental movies, mostly French and Italian, are shown is a joy. A 1946 French film has taken three years to reach the city, Jean Cocteau's romantic and surreal La Belle et la Bète (Beauty and the Beast). Out of the fairytale Cocteau spins a web of evocative illusion, placed in a mystical setting, the interior of a silent, threatening castle created with clever lighting, softly billowing curtains and wax-encrusted candlesticks, where a tragic lonely beast and a frightened beauty find love.

Fin flickers on the black screen; the house lights dimly glow and slowly intensify; and music filled with the sound of accordions swells as the auditorium empties. I file out with the crowd, jolted back into the real world but wanting to stay within the fairytale visited in the past hours.

Slipping between the circling glass panels, following the flow and stepping out of the revolving door into the foyer of the most elegant restaurant in the Cahill's chain, a thick floral carpet cushions my feet. Orange and yellow gladioli, arranged on the walnut counter, are reflected in the mirrored wall. The wide staircase leads up to the next floor, where dark-panelled walls, solid furniture and thickly padded banquettes are cosily ranged around the walls. This is my favoured room, rather than the downstairs section. Being alone I resist the head waitress's direction to take a seat that puts my back to the room, and I stand my ground in order to sit where I can face the room and observe the other patrons. This is one of the interesting aspects of city life. I cannot resist the caramel ice-cream cake, one of the restaurant's specialities: ice-cream is wedged between two layers of sponge cake and drenched in the thickest of caramel sauces.

My earlier steps down Martin Place in the direction of the Savoy Theatre had been taken eagerly. My return is set at a dawdling pace, pausing to stare into shop windows in a half-dreamy state, still in the land of Jean Cocteau. Reaching the hospital gates the bubble bursts and my stomach performs the usual acrobatic flip over.

'I always have that feeling too,' is Barbara's answer, later coming off duty and flopping onto the adjacent bed, when I reveal the emotions that surface every time I return to the hospital.

'I wonder if it will be a permanent reaction?' Dark circles are prominent beneath her eyes.

'I've had an awful day, so busy and never seeming to be able to please Sister—raising her voice to everyone to the point of shouting and putting everyone on edge. The atmosphere was dreadful.'

Many Sisters-in-charge and a few senior nurses have a reputation for this type of controlling bad-tempered supervision, and when trainees change wards we know what we have to expect when we have to confront a dragon. I'm not sure whether this goes hand in hand with nursing or is already there waiting for the right time and occupation in order to surface. Luckily I have not been the object of verbal abuse and hope to continue avoiding it.

Barbara finds some consolation in the wisdom passed on by the kindly Roman Catholic priest who knows the hospital well, and observes the progress of patients and staff, and the hurdles that need to be overcome by all. He always stops to enquire about her welfare.

An enclosed hospital community is like a small country town where news travels swiftly via the human telegraph and if you don't know the subject personally, then you know them by sight. Two nurses I can place by name, but with whom I have never worked, leave their training within a short space of time and under different circumstances.

Nurse Smithson, a quiet, retiring, second-year trainee, began to rapidly put on weight, her abdomen swelling until her predicament could no longer be overlooked by Matron. She has disappeared suddenly without explanation, with no goodbyes to anyone. She was close to bringing new life into the world, illegitimate, which is regarded as shameful, but she is also looked on with pity.

The second nurse ends a life by taking her own. A lonely death inflicted in a most painful way, she is found with a Lysol bottle beside her body, her alimentary tract excruciatingly consumed by a caustic agent commonly used around the hospital for cleaning and disinfection. Speculation is rife as to the reasons for her state of mind and the hospital telegraph hums once more, but in hushed tones.

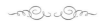

'A thief has stolen my best shoes.'

I stand, feeling on edge after searching the bedside table's lower shelf, where the footwear has been stored. No sign of the recent purchase. Flustered, I begin to rifle through my wardrobe, hauling the contents out onto the floor. No new cardboard shoebox to be found in the hanging section or in the drawers, dragged out and emptied, although it is most unlikely that even something as small as a handkerchief could have been squeezed into the already overflowing compartments.

'Has anyone borrowed them?'

Turning to face my roommates, all are present and resting on their beds. Seeing the surprised expression on each face of course it is a stupid, doubting question. Not one of them would borrow brand new shoes without permission. Over past pay days I have put aside an amount until I could purchase a pair of crisp, white, high-heeled ankle-strap sandals, crafted from finest leather, the band fitting across the instep decorated with lines of tiny punched out holes, the stilt heels a delight to behold.

The pleasurable aspects of residing in the best part of town are many, but living under institutionalised conditions has its drawbacks. In the sizable group of a shared environment, it is almost certain envy might cause a thief to make a move. No-one will dare wear my shoes within hospital precincts. Nevertheless, over coming weeks I will scrutinise the feet of any nurse on the point of going out dressed in street wear.

I will never see my expensive Italian footwear again, but it doesn't deter me from the pastime I cherish—and just ten minutes away—shopping for clothes.

6
Christmas Play

Ropes of tinsel twisted from wall to opposite wall, stirring lightly in the warm early morning breeze entering the opened upper windows; crepe paper, Christmas green and red, intermittently hung with coloured glass balls, is looped across bedheads. A cluster of pseudo-mistletoe swings above the entrance doorway, an added touch placed by an optimistic resident doctor hoping to catch the nurse of his choice passing beneath. I'm sure most will have reciprocal thoughts. After all, this is the season of festivity. I wonder whether Sister Bridgeman has noticed or realised the significance of this decoration.

Sister Lileblad is on the veranda, her white veil bobbing behind bowls of flowers arranged according to her decorative flair—not a drop spilled on her pristine uniform. The first task in Sister's morning is attractive and feminine—so unlike mine as I head towards pan room duty, where I will emerge with an apron spattered by undesirable stains. Someone has misplaced the rubber apron again.

If caught and kissed beneath the mistletoe by one of the young residents maybe Sister's perfect assurance will slip a little, the expression on her smooth face might show some emotion. This ward is her show, a daily performance and she is the stage manager, Christmas or otherwise, supervising all the characters acting out their roles, in an hour-by-hour presentation. She corrects any break in continuity, controls added drama, eliminates lapses in the staged routine of every day, and sets right misplaced timings.

Working in the wings, not waiting on cue to enter and fill an important role, I remain in lowly status scrubbing bed pans and swilling out unpleasant clinging residue. Urinals and sputum mugs are cleaned and polished, and the latter's slimy cardboard inserts replaced with fresh. All of these indispensable props are loaded in and out of the pan steriliser with bulky, purpose-built forceps, and with a clanging of gleaming metal they are displayed in horizontal rows on the racks provided. Now where is the thrill of nervous excitement I had felt on my first day while looking out of my bedroom window and sighting a white veil or doctor's coat?

St Mary's Cathedral, positioned in such close proximity to the hospital, resonates with changes rung out across the city. The sound of peals, entering through the south-facing windows, glorifies the day and the ward. The imagined bell-ringers, tugging down on their ropes in succession then riding up off the floor, make me feel uplifted too; my thoughts turn towards home and how Christmas Day might be progressing. The sound of family voices yesterday, Christmas Eve, was comforting after standing in a long queue before placing my telephone call at the GPO. I check my watch. Mother, Father and sister Annette will be with friends by now. Later, circled around the festive table, pulling bonbons, they will exchange the jokes found inside, crown themselves with a gaudy crepe paper hat, eat too much and return home for an afternoon nap—Dad snoring rowdily on his back; Mum breathing more delicately by his side.

Another glance at the ward clock quickens my pace. There are beds to carbolise, vacated by patients discharged earlier. The mattresses are swabbed with a diluted solution of carbolic or

Lysol, then dragged out to the veranda to air on the mattress rack. Bed frame, locker, bed table and bed cradle are swabbed. Fresh mattresses are hoisted inside and beds made up for the next admissions.

Ward 5, that fragment in the theatre of life, has many cast changes, but some characters remain much longer than others. Passing down the line of beds, serving the usual mid-morning drinks from my trolley, I pause at the foot of Mr Rosenthal's bed, placed in an area adjacent to the desk. He has suffered a coronary occlusion (myocardial infarction)—a heart attacked caused by the blockage of a cardiac artery—and must have complete bed rest and, in order to aid nature's healing process, absolute physical and mental rest from emotional strain. For several weeks, or as determined by his Honorary Physician, he must not make any unassisted movement, so he is treated as a 'helpless patient'. He is fed, lifted on and off the pan, sponged, teeth cleaned and only later is he permitted to gradually regain movement, the absolute immobility ordered initially with the intention of preventing the clot from moving and threatening the blood supply to his heart. He sucks the juice from the feeding cup while I hold the utensil chatting about nothing and wishing I could stay longer. He is an uncomplaining patient, the latter word being the operative one in his case.

Mr Marksworth's complaint, a descriptive noun surely created for him, is pericarditis (inflammation of the heart's outer lining) and he is nursed under the same conditions. For pain, morphine injections or Dovers Pulv. (powder) 15 gr is administered, depending on the severity. Occasionally a warm starch poultice is applied to his left upper chest to ease the discomfort. The No. 7 Indispensable Quality Desirable in a Nurse is rolled into one, but sympathy, tact and understanding are applied with effort to Mr Marksworth, who doesn't deal successfully with illness and whose reactions to most attentions and requests are anger, irritability and rudeness.

Mr Green is another facing a long stay, sitting beside his bed observing me with a melancholic expression covering his gaunt face, the typical presentation of someone diagnosed with a duodenal ulcer. Caused by excess stress and hyperacidity affecting the stomach's lining, he has little to be pleased about as the Yuletide mealtime draws nearer. His mournful eyes gaze on a glass of milk placed on his bed table and, turning up his nose, forces a wan smile. 'Fluids only' is the instruction on his bedhead and the beginning of a regime known as a 'Sippy Diet'. Administered in consultation with the dietician and consisting of second hourly nourishment, milk drinks or creamy eggnog, the amounts are increased weekly. Other milk-based foods will be gradually introduced, until a light diet is allowed in perhaps four to six weeks.

The simple task of handing the appropriate drink to each patient should not have lethal consequences, but hearing Janet recount her experience in serving sugar-laced orange juice to several diabetic patients is a reminder not to lose concentration in even the simplest tasks. Realising her mistake and reporting it to her ward sister, Sister Lileblad's antithesis, a storm blew up in the middle of the ward. Feared because of her reputation and fierce pug-like countenance, Sister shouted abuse and dressed Janet down, circled by a grandstand of astonished patients. The RMO was summoned to keep a check on the patients' blood sugar and later, when all had settled down, he left, giving a nonplussed Janet, being as pretty as she is, a friendly, forgiving grin.

Patients fit to consume a normal diet are pleased with the extra effort bestowed on Christmas dinner by the kitchen staff and the creation of a festive atmosphere. They have partly achieved that themselves, with Sister persisting in her efforts to teach some patients the art of cutting crepe paper and the production of decorations.

Sister avoids being caught and kissed beneath the mistletoe

and therefore loses none of her equanimity. My passing beneath the ward entrance archway never coincides with that of an approaching male. I feel slightly disappointed. Those with outgoing personalities, mainly Senior Nurses, make sure they are standing under the white berries of the mistletoe just as a good-natured doctor arrives or exits.

We sample leftover chicken and roast vegetables behind the day room door while Sister is at lunch. Chicken, a luxury served only at Christmas, is on the menu every Sunday in the resident doctors' dining room, though we hold no grudge against the 33 RMOs for this privilege. Being on call isn't easy. Their work shifts are arduous and long, and their tired brains are pushed to make life and death decisions.

A modern paging system has been installed in each ward foyer near the ward telephone. A pale grey screen is suspended from the high ceiling, blinking with an array of numbers. This requires the constant attention of medical and top nursing staff passing through the hospital watching for his or her assigned number. If that appears the switchboard is immediately contacted.

This is my first Christmas Day spent away from home. I dare not dwell on it and will be glad when this shift has ended. Perhaps the other country girls, Judy and Dulcie, will be somewhere in the Nightingale Wing, and I check the ward clock again.

7
New Year, New Decade

The climb back to our room after breakfast follows the slant of the cedar staircase, a grand internal construction built in the centre of the Nightingale Wing, connecting the floors from the lower ground to the fourth, which had been added in 1895. The solid balustrade held within my grip, fingers slipping up the polished patina of wood feels like satin. Opening the door to our room, the striking nineteenth-century features in wood, which do not extend beyond the doorway, are a great contrast to this bleak interior and the complete lack of decoration or comfort. Perhaps the accommodation will improve on graduation; the Sisters' Sitting Room, glimpsed through an open doorway, reveals chintz-covered chairs and silver on the table set for tea. Afternoon tea is surely taken with the best of manners.

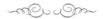

The morning is free after breakfast and we must decide how to fill in the hours. Flopping onto her bed Janet releases a long sigh. It is best to avoid the stiff, hard-backed chair allotted to each bed and not meant for relaxation.

'Here it is, 1950 and I will be 20 this year. I can't believe I am that old already.' Adding before I can reply, 'You may not think so but I'm not entirely sure that where I'm heading is the right choice.'

'I suggest that we should head for downtown and spend a few hours exploring our favourite shopping arcade.'

Janet's face rarely looks solemn and now lights up. Forgetting that life is rapidly passing her by she replies, 'I can't think of a more pleasant way in which to spend the morning.'

We change and I broach the subject again. 'I think it quite likely that all of us will feel restless at times. Why did you choose nursing?'

Janet, pulling on a nylon stocking and fastening it to her suspender, turns to check the back seam in the mirror to make sure the line running down the back of her calf is straight. She is notorious for wearing crooked seams and I point out that the left is way off-centre.

'My parents encouraged me and my father kept insisting what a noble profession it is. But my intention now is to become an air hostess and travel. A nursing diploma is a great asset when applying, but the thought of ploughing through four years here is, at this moment, daunting.'

Maybe she is still smarting from the confrontation over the hazardous sugar additive to the orange juice. With her sweet personality and ability to remain calm under most circumstances, I can visualise her looking smartly confident in the dark tailored uniform and peak cap of an air hostess.

'Then you do have a positive goal,' I said. 'Whatever happens, I am sure it will work out.'

How fortunate Janet is in having gained the end of school Leaving Certificate. And her parents' home is in the city, where there are choices and advantages when choosing a career.

I select my smartest outfit, plus matching hat, gloves, handbag and shoes, hoping to feel one with the crowd while browsing through the area, part laneway and part arcade, running from

Castlereagh Street down to Pitt Street. The cosy pedestrian thoroughfare known as Rowe Street is a pleasant enclave, a place where we can indulge ourselves gazing in shop windows, and watching the parade of stylish men and women.

The tiny shops are stocked with luxury goods. The mix of fashion, art and literature, including avant-garde pictures and banned books, has been compared with Paris and I cannot dispute this, not having the experience to doubt those who travel to that great city on the other side of the world.

One of the swinging signs hanging above the shops reads 'Henriette Lamotte'. A milliner who has studied in Paris, her salon is decorated with gilded sofas covered in ocelot fur and most of her merchandise, chic hats and accessories, are imported from France. Fabulous buttons and ornaments, hand-made blouses, elegant scarves displayed in other shops make window shopping exciting as we point to beautiful items we adore but just can't afford.

Marion Best, interior designer, stocks imported goods from Scandinavia and Japan, displayed beneath clever lighting. Much admired are the Swedish glass and the Marimekko fabrics from Finland with modern designs like nothing I have seen before.

This fascination with unattainable items and places extends to rooms above street level. These areas I doubt I will ever see but I remain curious. Looking up at the windows I imagine the passage of light filtering into the artists' and writers' garret studios or dance and ballet schools. A world away from the rooms and wards where we learn our skills.

It is the second day of a new decade and a new look in fashion: narrow belted waists, long full skirts, black high-heeled suede shoes and stunning hats. The New Look is worn by so many passing women moving into or coming from Henriette Lamotte or the Hotel Australia at the top end of the lane.

By 1973 Rowe Street will be gone forever, following demolition of the Hotel Australia. Cut in two, the Castlereagh Street end of Rowe Street will be absorbed into a new structure, the MLC Centre. For anyone who knew the small unique area it is remembered with fondness—and sadness for the loss of those very special shops.

Sitting in a Rowe Street coffee shop, observing this city haunt of those who love a cosmopolitan atmosphere and feeling one of them, I try to make it a diversion, hoping my coffee will drown the butterflies coming to life and beating their wings on my stomach wall. These pulsating creatures react like an alarm set to warn when a shift is imminent.

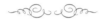

Moving on to another ward is a daunting prospect. Our studies have changed from medical to surgical nursing, and so our wards change too.

The door shuttles sideways and I step into the ancient lift, purpose-built to carry the variable loads that are shunted around a hospital—staff, visitors, trolleys, beds, wheelchairs and stacked provisions. The lift attendant pushes the door into position, gives a robust pull on the thick rope running down through the roof and out through the floor. The ride up is quite smooth but comes to a halt with a jerk and several unexpected bounces.

Ward 16 is of the customary open design, divided into two ends, male and female, by a foyer containing the lift well, Sister's office and the day room. The Travers Building that houses the surgical wards, built in 1930, is situated at the rear of the hospital grounds bordering the Domain. Its a rectangular block lacking the architectural imagination demonstrated in the original buildings at the front of the site.

The views from the upper floors of Travers looking over the harbour and city are magnificent—when one can afford time to stop and appreciate the vista.

My confidence has been fortified a fraction in the knowledge that Sister Dempsey, sister-in-charge, is not a member of the dragon brigade but one who supervises an efficient ward firmly and fairly. I learned this from Barbara's mother, Mrs Quinlan, who is Sister Dempsey's close friend and neighbour and tells us about Dempsey's experience as a probationer while training at the hospital in tougher times.

Under Matron Kellett's reign, the previous matron of 20-years' standing, who had a fierce reputation, Sister Dempsey sought permission to attend her brother's funeral and requested a day of compassionate leave. This was granted on one condition: that after the funeral she forego the wake and return immediately to duty. Grief for her brother's loss and her family's state on the day and her own emotional upheaval made it clear she must remain with them. Returning the following day, she would have been summoned into Matron's office and was told she must repeat the length of time in training already completed, almost 12 months, and begin again from that day of reprimand.

Surgical nursing is more interesting. There are more patients of a younger age and most stay in hospital for several weeks after surgical procedures. Young men admitted with a condition requiring a simpler operation, such as acute appendicitis, are sometimes cheeky, checking my name badge and entreating me to tell them my first name. It is better not to reveal this and pass it off good-naturedly. Armed with this knowledge some will go too far, grinning broadly, passing the name on in a loud voice so that others in the ward catch on and treat this information as everyone's business. This wouldn't please Sister. The rule is that staff should not be addressed by first names as a sign of respect and good manners. But Sister doesn't hear the soft wolf whistle directed at me and I feel flattered, responding with a grin.

My first introduction to Mr Wangensteen's Apparatus occurs the following week. I assume Wangensteen is or was a medico referred to as 'Mr' in the tradition of reference given to honorary surgeons who attend public patients free of charge. This invention's design is similar to the moving comic sculptures of the artist Heath Robinson, but it brings no comic relief to the patient. Its similarity is in its simplicity.

Its purpose is to provide a continuous gastric siphonage that works in a simple way to produce negative or positive pressure at will and flushes out the stomach contents following gastric surgery. I pity the solitary night nurse responsible for overseeing this apparatus, with the constant supervision necessary while attending to everyone else's needs. Six months' ward experience, including the time spent in Tutor School, and I will soon be one of those solitary care-givers of the night.

8
Toil by Torchlight

The lamp Florence Nightingale carried in the Crimean War became her symbol so that she was named for posterity the 'Lady with the Lamp'. Our night duty hours are lit by a square metal box with the bulb positioned in front and a handle on top. It is designed to sit safely on a bedside surface and has no comparison with illustrations of the Aladdin-style oil lamp Florence Nightingale carried in the Crimea. The lamp synonymous with her story offered minimal safety, with the tiny bare flame glowing on top and held perilously close to her voluminous skirts—perhaps it was the only type available in the Crimea. My lamp will not cause a fire but in case of that dreaded catastrophe occurring, I decide I should check how many fire extinguishers are hanging on their hooks in Ward 15 where I have been assigned.

Dr Norman Rose, Medical Superintendent, on his nightly midnight round accompanied by the Night Sister, will stand at the ward entrance and throw questions at me and expect me to know the answers about equipment as well as patients.

Less than 12 hours' notice has been given for transfer to night duty. At ten o'clock this morning, while on duty in Ward 16, Sister called me to her office.

'Matron's office wishes to speak to you,' and I feel weak at the knees. I scold myself on the way to the phone: I must learn to accept change in a smarter way. Lifting the receiver, I quake again, for Matron Pidgeon is personally instructing me to go off duty and report for night duty that evening. In the meantime I must move, bag and baggage, out of the Nightingale Wing to the night nurses' quarters on the top floor of Sydney Eye Hospital in Woolloomooloo.

Another room of desolate proportions with blinds inefficient for blocking out daylight. After lunch and unpacking, I lie on the creaky bed. Sleep, which might have fortified me for the coming night, is kept at bay by a feeling of inadequacy and fear of not coping, which precedes any looming unknown task. Negative thinking, I chide myself—I haven't failed yet.

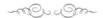

Together Barbara and I select our torches from the table where they are set out near the bundy clock that records our hours on the ward. The machine sucks the card from my hand and marks the time with a heavy clang. We set out at a fast trot across the darkened courtyard towards the Travers Building and Ward 15 for, with a great stroke of luck, we are working together. Barbara will care for the female patients and I for the males as the ward plan is the same as Ward 16 above. Within calling distance of each other, with only the entrance foyer in between, I will be able to look across the space and see the glow from my friend's torch moving down the row of beds or see her sitting at the desk, a faint shadow behind the lowered desk lamp.

Clutching our blue waist-length capes closer around the chest, we hurry up the stairs winding around the lift well. The lift rests quietly in its cage on the ground floor, unattended in the night hours. Shoes kicked off in the change room, feet clad in brand new slippers, cuffs discarded on the shelves, we approach Sister's Office. The Senior Nurse is waiting to run through the afternoon/

evening report on both male and female sections so that together we will know every patient's diagnosis and condition.

A quick ward round led by the Senior Nurse and we pause before the more seriously ill. Beneath torchlight aimed at the bedhead and not into the patient's face she whispers instructions. The grotesque sound of someone struggling for breath is unmistakable, issuing out of the gloom midway down the ward on the opposite side. We cross over to that area and in the shallow torchlight a patient in his middle years is revealed, propped high up in a Fowler's position, a chair-like arrangement of pillows. His forehead is glistening with sweat and stringy saliva mixed with viscous phlegm is frothing out of the artificial aperture in the base of his throat.

'It's quite simple to clear the tracheostomy cannula,' the Senior Nurse states calmly. I am sure she has noted my startled expression in the ghostly lighting around the bed, and on the opposite side Barbara's ashen face. Although we have witnessed disturbing sights and unsavoury treatments, as novices in a darkened ward coupled with sole responsibility, everything seems doubly intense. As yet I stand in awe of senior nurses, admiring their confidence and knowledge gained by the third and fourth year of training and the power attained; how they sweep ahead through a doorway, their starched apron tails flapping with vigour while we, the untried, stand aside.

Confidently the nurse demonstrates the simplicity of easing the patient's distress. Uncovering the bedside tray, removing the rubber catheter from a kidney dish, the suction pump is turned on and the attached catheter is introduced into the yellow white substance oozing out of his trachea. She shows caution in how far to introduce the suction as sludge moves swiftly past the window provided by a glass connection in the rubber tubing.

'What if the catheter becomes blocked?' I ask, voicing the worst of many disastrous scenarios pelting through my brain, forcing myself to concentrate, because very soon this confident senior is going to vanish down the stairwell and into the night. She explains how the suction of normal saline drawn from a bowl placed on the tray will clear the blockage and she adds an afterthought: 'Remember to call the Senior Night Nurse if you have any difficulty.'

My optimism is now on the rise. Suddenly concern for myself and my ability is transferred to Mr Hunter, the patient who must bear with the unnatural fluid eruptions emerging from the dark hole in his neck, his speech taken away and replaced by the inability to communicate. The panic momentarily falls away. Mr Hunter is relying on me to see him through the night. I can look forward to a break, go to supper and inhale a comforting cigarette. There's no respite open to him and when I clock off in the morning he will remain without the luxury of choice that is mine in going or staying.

The first brilliant rays spread above the distant ocean then creep across the eastern seaboard. Macquarie Lighthouse on South Head is aflame with a fiery orange; the cheerful sound of day staff voices carrying ahead of their pounding footsteps up the stairwell are wonderful sights and sounds.

Mr Hunter and I survived the night. I have successfully answered Dr Rose's questioning, emptied pans and bottles, recorded fluid balance charts, charted temperatures, written my report, been sent to supper by the relieving night nurse, sponged several patients and placated those bereft of sleep due to Mr Hunter's noisy distress and the intermittent strident suction. Early morning tea, served by myself and several walking patients who are eager to assist, is over.

There has been no time to watch for Barbara's torch glow bobbing around her female patients at the other end. We did pass each other once or twice as I hurried into the day room to snatch a blanket out of the hot cupboard while Barbara was pulling ice cubes out of the refrigerator. These and many other duties have kept the soles of our woolly slippers burnishing the bare boards of Ward 15 for the past eight hours.

While waiting for the hospital car, which shuttles staff back and forth when going to or coming off duty to various quarters scattered out of the hospital's precincts, fatigue drops like a heavenly parachute. When reaching earth it billows out slowly and encompasses the weary beneath its canopy.

The car rounds the curve in St Mary's Road and there is a spontaneous groan from the occupants. Road repairs are underway in Sir John Young Crescent. A cacophony of jackhammers thundering, trucks grinding gears and labourers shouting rages directly below our night duty sleeping quarters.

This is a surreal existence, sleeping in daylight hours waking at 4 p.m., shuffling bleary-eyed to afternoon tea following sleep taken during unnatural hours, which never refreshes the body thoroughly. Free time has never passed so quickly.

One by one the others in the group are sent to join the night staff. The two months' duration is lightened by evening walks up poorly lit streets, though we always feel safe, to Kings Cross, mecca of Sydney night-life. We pass rows of shabby terraces offering glimpses of cramped interiors through open front doors, until we reach a burst of flashing neon lights and raucous nightclub spruikers, not fully in swing until we have to leave.

Returning downhill, the navy blue harbour is a splendid backdrop for illuminated ships moving east and west, creating lines of light that zigzag into Woolloomooloo Bay.

Hearing the throaty warning from a ship's horn makes it good to know others are on shift work too and keeping the city functioning.

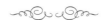

Rugged up in mid-winter, cocooned in the railway carriage, my feet rest cosily upon the lead foot warmer supplied by the New South Wales government railways. This overnight snug space is mine until Wauchope Station glides by the window and I alight for my destination, Port Macquarie. Meanwhile, with increased speed, the steel wheels below stomp along the track; my suitcase rocks in the metal luggage rack overhead; and the carriage sways, soothing as a cradle, shunting me in and out of sleep. Night duty is in the past. Four days off lie ahead, days that will gallop by before my return to day duty again. The steam engine gives a shrill whistle in celebration, pulling me on, ever closer to home.

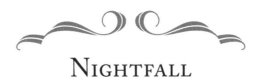

николай

Nightfall

Sleep—serenity ... *induced by shadowy darkness descending, have no place in the female ward where Nurse Elizabeth Morrow tends the needs of 20 patients through a long, weary night. Thirteen are afflicted by typhoid fever. Macquarie Street is a quiet thoroughfare after 10.00 p.m. The occasional carriage passes with clunking horses' hooves and squeaking harness fading away, the scant beam from carriage lights swallowed up in the gloom. Entering the eastern windows, the plaintive cry of an owl nesting in the Domain drifts in, then settles. These nightly sounds are out of tune with the internal cries of humans in pain, the believers beseeching God to free them from their misery.*

Nurse Morrow, a fetching Irish girl, knows this scene well, being one who has nursed Infirmary patients for some time before Miss Osburn's arrival and satisfactorily enough to be selected to stay. A tall girl with strong limbs and thick auburn hair that rebelliously falls from her cap, she seems to be endowed with unlimited physical strength.

The latest admission is calling out for a nurse and, reaching the bedside, Elizabeth drops her voice to a whisper, although the majority of patients seem to be awake. The exceptions, too weak now, are unable to raise a voice, asking for her attention.

'What is the matter, Mary?'

'I couldn't wait for the pot, Nurse,' and clutching at her lower abdomen, 'the pain, my God, the pain— here it comes again.' The liquid sound of bowel contents mixed with wind ruptures forth from the depths of the covering grey blanket.

Pulling back the bedclothes the nurse's hand brushes over Mary's limbs, heated as though on fire, and the smell is atrocious. If miasma is the cause of this persecution how will Elizabeth avoid this disease? She pushes the thought away, knowing that the foul smell from faulty drains are the source of disease, not the breathing in the odour from a filthy sheet. She has been told this by one who knows—the doctor in charge. Poor Mary's abdominal muscles are taut, pressing down, the bowel empty but straining to keep on purging, drawing precious body fluids into that canal and evacuating them.

Swiftly Elizabeth changes the underneath mattress covering, which is no more than a bundle of rags pushed beneath Mary's buttocks. The clean linen supply was exhausted an hour ago and whatever strips of sheeting can be found are substituted. Miss Osburn has already made some inroads in her short time here, attempting to solve this problem, she has fought the opposition received from Blackstone in his managerial position.

'I will bring your next dose of laudanum as soon as it's due.'

The narcotic painkiller, containing morphine and prepared from opium, gives relief, subduing the bowel contractions, but it wears off before the next dose is due. As Elizabeth gives this reassurance she gently strokes Mary's bald head. All the heads are shaved, helping to reduce the high temperature and encouraging a strong regrowth, as the hair tends to fall out following a fever. This practice also helps control head lice.

There is scant time available to spend on each patient. Ideally, at intervals, she should drizzle cold water over feverish limbs, trying not to saturate the mattress, and if time allows she manages to treat a few.

Fever parches the throat and hoarsens the voice. Holding the feeding cup in position above Maggie's mouth, dripping a few drops from the spout onto her cracked lips Nurse Morrow tries to encourage the young woman to swallow.

'Open your mouth Maggie.' She gives praise in her musical Irish brogue when a few sips are taken.

'Good girl, Maggie. Don't you worry my darlin', the Lord will bring *this to an end and you will be your old self again.'*

She pulls the pan out from beneath the bedclothes and in a fast trot covers the ward's length and enters a side room.

Full buckets of body residue stand in a row and when the lids are lifted, a covering insisted on by Miss Osburn, the same foul smell of dirty beds is released. This is the salvaged filth able to be caught in time and ready for disposal.

A bucket in each hand Elizabeth has no choice but to leave the ward. The pad of her feet thrums on bare boards through the passage of several wards before reaching the one toilet provided for 50 patients.

'Things will change.' Miss Osburn had been appalled seeing the state of sanitation, or lack of it, on her arrival. She also questions the practice of leaving a nurse in the same difficult ward for too long, especially on night duty.

'No wonder she becomes bad-tempered with failing health. Should one stay up all night for three years? No!' she expostulates.

Returning quickly and before she can replace her empty buckets, Elizabeth is greeted by a wailing and sobbing set off by two patients near the door, fearing they had been abandoned when Elizabeth vanished through the entrance. Seeing her reappear those fears are banished and the crying ceases.

Replacing the emptied vessels Elizabeth quickly pours stored water from a jug into an enamel basin and washes her hands, working up a lather, rubbing the suds firmly into her skin. She knows this should be done more often but is not achieved due to her workload. Miss Osburn has been very insistent on the importance of cleanliness as taught in the Nightingale system of nursing, but it's not easy to initiate in wards without taps or basins. The Sisters have also insisted and supervised practices of scrubbing; the changing face of some areas emerging from a scene of squalor.

New techniques of wound care are being gradually accepted and practised more widely with good results, such as dressings soaked in a carbolic acid solution inserted into or covering wounds. The proof that *bacteria exist and cause disease and infection is still ten years away.*

5.00 a.m.

Another hour and Nurse Elizabeth Morrow will be relieved. Two more nights and she will move onto day duty. Her drooping eyelids and aching limbs are calling out for rest. The physical exertion of the previous hours has brought on a pounding headache. A pain so intense it is boring into her skull behind her nose, spreading into her cheekbones and affecting her vision. Cold shivers shake her body, her forehead is feverish to the touch. The sudden onset of spasmodic pain is as sharp as a dagger being plunged into her abdomen and her rectum is on fire. She rushes towards the side room, whips her uniform up around her waist, releases her bloomers and the repugnant liquid explodes out of her squatting body into the waiting bucket.

9

The Straw and the Camel's Back

The train engine belches a last whiff of coal-fired soot, and discharges a final defiant hiss of steam between resting wheels as I alight onto the platform at Central Station. Inviting me back on this crisp autumn morning Sydney is waiting, revealing how splendid she can look. I hurry towards the tram stop, across the open space of parkland swathed in early morning sun. Dew is dissolving on the grass; the cool light sharpens building outlines.

The same old room in the Nightingale Wing also waits, with its lack of heating, antiquated worn furniture disguised by pallid lighting, a residence that might be renamed Bleak House. Muffled conversation is heard in the corridor before the door bursts open and Pat enters the room uttering her usual deep mirthful chuckle.

'You're back, how lovely to see you and sharing a room, great.' Removing her cap and kicking off her shoes she continues, 'My poor feet—they are crying out for some pampering.'

Plonking down on the bed beside me she begins to massage her stockinged toes.

'Next time our days off coincide you must come home with me, Gran loves having you stay the night.'

Joined by Barbara bustling in, her violin case deposited in the bottom of her wardrobe, she is looking flushed after a quick walk up Martin Place from her violin lesson at a music studio near Wynyard. She too is relieved to be back on day duty, and chattering ceaselessly we change into uniform.

Having worked through *Sears Anatomy and Physiology* cover to cover, a small volume in comparison with *Gray's Anatomy*, the weighty tome seen in the hands of medical students, lectures on that subject are finished. Several had fallen on afternoons during night duty, which meant rising earlier from the day's sleep to attend. The same compulsory attendance applies should lectures be held during the fortnightly two nights off, and I am given leave from the ward on this afternoon's shift to attend another teaching hour: ear, nose and throat nursing.

A book placed beside the bundy clock sets out staff ward changes and new placements; my name is marked beside Ward 2, a female medical ward situated on the first floor in one of the original front buildings. Sister Glasson is in charge, tall, slim, freckled face and thankfully graced with a reasonable disposition despite her red hair. Once I have reported to her and been excused after the reading of the report, I retrace my steps, quickly negotiating the flight of stairs leading to the ground floor and Outpatients. My group is already gathered around a patient sitting in one of the cubicles. The Ear, Nose and Throat Registrar is seated too, facing a young man. Standing to one side a nurse is assisting, holding a kidney dish beneath the patient's chin, a rubber cape is draped over his shoulder. The Registrar explains the treatment as he proceeds. First one nasal passage is dealt with then the other.

Standing around such a patient, who in a public teaching hospital can be subjected to group observation, I feel uncomfortable for the young man as though we are voyeurs, particularly as the treatment is verging very quickly on the invasive.

Local anaesthetic on a cotton swab is inserted in each nostril, left to take effect and removed. A thin metal cannula is inserted and forced into the sinus cavity with a horrifying crunch of pierced bone. I wince, my toes squirm in my shoes and my palms are sweaty. The young man does not appear to be suffering any pain but his pupils are enlarged and glassy as he tries to grab at the instrument lodged in his nasal passage. The assistant nurse quickly instructs Pat to hold his hands. A syringe is attached to the cannula and the sinus cavity irrigated with normal saline, dislodging copious gluey slime into the kidney dish. The force applied, the accompanying crack of breaking bone ensures that both he and I will never forget that sound. For me there is an added memory, the combined ghostly pallor and distressed expression on his face.

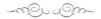

I take the steps two at a time, report to Sister Glasson then move to assist in turning Mrs Sharp, a mother with small children and a long-time patient in Ward 2. She is afflicted with disseminated sclerosis (a disease causing widespread hardening and contraction of muscle tissue), her miseries are multiple, and her worst ordeal is due to our essential constant caring attention: the second hourly changing position, washing and skincare of her back and pressure points. Just to touch her skin seems to be agonising. Turning her is worse despite sedation. A hell on earth, which she suffers with stoicism.

A daily strict record is kept in every ward. The 'back book' lists the condition of bed patients' pressure points and is presented at Matron's office every morning, then checked and signed by her. Bedsores are an anathema and Matron is the first to denunciate their development.

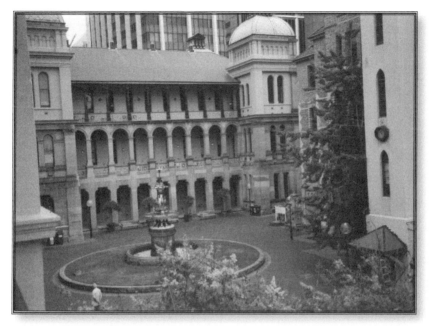

Sydney Hospital, 2008. In 1950 facing wards were Ground Floor—Outpatients; First Floor—Ward 2; Second Floor—Ward 3. (Author photograph)

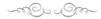

The dress gently unfolds as I lift it from the hastily opened parcel; brown paper and layers of tissue scatter to the floor. I hold the soft wool up against my body, turning to study the mirror's reflection. This is the eagerly awaited finished product sewn by my mother from a dress length purchased before my brief visit home after night duty. The memory of that visit comes flooding back.

My mother's dressmaker's scissors have sliced assuredly around the pattern edge and through the sky blue wool laid out on the kitchen table, a line of pins stuck in her cardigan cuff were deftly plucked out and placed in her work. I have no interest in sewing, so it looks like a jigsaw puzzle to me. Peddling confidently, feeding the material beneath the needle's rapid movement, my mother and her Singer sewing machine have brought it all together. I spread the finished handiwork across the bed. I admire the raglan sleeves and lay my wide brown suede belt peppered with chrome studs across the waistline, and for full effect place near the hemline my brown and white pumps—sought and found after much browsing through shoe shops.

There is no time to linger or try the dress on. Due to relieve in Ward 8 this afternoon, and for the coming week temporarily bypassing Ward 2, I quickly change and make my way to the building opposite the Nightingale Wing. The top floor houses the hospital's only children's ward.

Walking into Ward 8 I am left in no doubt how busy or thoroughly noisy the coming week will be or how, now and then, all will intensify as though bedlam has broken out. Hit by a blast of vigorous shouting and crying in varying depths of tone, little people sit on their pillows or stand at the end of cots ranged down each side of the open space. Mouths are contorted into a wide aperture, demanding attention. A few too ill to fuss lie quietly, neatly tucked in and barely discernable behind the cot sides. The child who rules the ward due to his long hospitalisation makes an impression on all who come and go. Everyone has to pass his cot, first on the left when entering, where he hangs over the end rattling the bars, stamping his feet on the mattress, deprived of speech, air whistling in or spluttering out of his tracheostomy; a legacy of swallowing a screw that lodged in his throat and was removed with difficulty. He faces further surgery and a lengthy stay. Little Kenny Elder is about two years of age and, even when his tactics alter and he quietens, making an attempt to whimper and hold out his arms, puts some fear into my heart. Experience with babies is foreign to me, except with my sister who is still very young, three years old when I left home. I survive the week guided by the one in charge, Sister Blue, a tall statuesque blonde never ruffled by those in her care.

Kenny's equivalent in an adult patient, drawing attention and refusing to follow reasonable requests, is Bea Miles. Kenny, child that he is, must eventually comply, Bea never. She merely ignores instructions or requests of any kind, another patient I regard with awe after our paths cross in Ward 16. Once a member of a family of wealthy Sydney merchants, Bea took on the role of vagrant and is now known to everyone around town, a bane to police and especially taxi drivers, jumping into cabs then vociferously refusing to pay. The cabbies are no match for Bea. A common sight in the streets, driving like the queen of the city, her barrel shape is clothed in a dress riding above her knees; her accessories are a sunshade, sandshoes and a shoulder-strap canvas bag.

She does her own thing in Ward 16, taking leave to go down town, or maybe for a taxi ride, and returning at will. Between times she shows an unexpected talent as a knowledgeable exponent of the works of William Shakespeare, acquired at university. Discharged from hospital to return to her nightly abode in a culvert, she doesn't part company with staff altogether. Periodically revisiting the ward, she washes out her matronly bloomers in the day room sink, then places them to dry on the hot table. While waiting, she consumes a leftover midday meal offered by Sister, who understands that remonstrating with her never works and only serves to make her aggressive. No-one classifies Bea as mentally unstable. Patients diagnosed as unstable are sent as inpatients to specialist psychiatric institutions such as Callan Park and Broughton Hall.

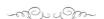

Our first year of training is almost complete and mornings are now warmer when we have to rise early; the initial contact of toes on linoleum does not cause the reaction of quickly withdrawing the feet back under the warm bedclothes. Pulling the rest of my body into a standing position I lean across to give the alarm clock a sharp whack. I do not have the refreshed feeling that a good night's sleep brings. A late shift followed by a morning one means working 2 p.m. until 10 p.m. then taking time to settle into sleep, usually not before midnight, the day's events surging through my mind. Up again at 5 a.m. for duty at six I feel physically drained and the waiting workload in Ward 2 is heavy.

A feeling of envy emerges when I think of my easygoing, friends Dulcie and Judy, who have resigned. They leave in three weeks to resume country life in their respective home towns. They yearn for the free and healthy lifestyle with boyfriends left behind, and marriage is decidedly a part of the future.

Janet is certain she will leave midway into the following year and travel by sea to Great Britain with her parents. Her aim of becoming an air hostess hasn't waned and she is intending to apply to British Overseas Airways Corporation (BOAC) hoping two years' nursing experience will be a suitable qualification. Mr Burstal is troubled by his daughter's decision not to finish her training, but he needs to requite his passion for all things British and not postpone his visit. The thought of losing Janet's company and the effect her endearing personality has on the group makes me feel restless.

Attention to patients' hygiene and bedmaking complete, at least for the early part of the day, the ward is swept. Sister Bridgeman's round is over, taking with her the pointing, accusing finger that detects various out-of-place objects offensive to her Deputy Matron's senses. Placing the thermometer tray on the bed table, a vigorous flick to shake down the mercury, I misjudge the distance. My hand-eye co-ordination is sometimes poor and the reason why I am a hopeless tennis player. The glass thermometer snaps into several pieces, silver pearls of mercury, almost impossible to recapture, roll across the metal surface of the bed table.

A visit to Matron's office is routine for such carelessness. An explanation is obligatory before a replacement is given.

The salvaged pieces of glass in one hand, I tap tentatively on Matron's office door. A voice instructs me to enter and I step across the threshold. Not sure what my next move should be,

I feel awkward standing beside the desk, my hands clasped dutifully behind my back. Matron doesn't cease her writing or lift her head. She is seated on a sturdy cedar chair behind a wide, impressive desk, also built from cedar. Both pieces are superb examples of early colonial furniture and were ordered by Lucy Osburn. Manufactured by the firm of Joseph Raphael they have been used by each succeeding Matron.

The atmosphere is hushed except for the occasional clink of cutlery on crockery in the next room as Matron's maid bustles in and out from the adjoining pantry setting her lunch table, and the scratching of Matron's fountain pen rapidly moving across paper.

'Yes, Nurse?' At last Matron speaks.

'I am requesting a replacement thermometer, Matron.'

Without a pause in attending to her copious paperwork Matron's reply is the surprise manifestation of a lecture and must be boringly repetitious for her.

'Carelessness on your part is a cost to the hospital budget. Every broken item replaced is usually caused by lack of concentration and could have been avoided. In future be more careful, Nurse. Add your name into the thermometer register and sign your name.'

There was no acceptable excuse and that is obvious, so why attempt one, but I feel a flush heating my face. I cannot remember being reprimanded, certainly not at school where I recall only being praised. No. 8 Indispensable Quality Desirable in a Nurse is Economy, and in this respect I have failed.

Lucy Osburn and Rose Creal, Matron from 1898 to 1921 and another revered personage, regally photographed and framed, hang on opposite walls, their faint smiles and knowing looks seem to indicate that they had endured the same incompetency in their day, from clumsy girls with no thoughts on the necessity of economy.

I hope Matron will raise her head and identify me by name, acknowledge I am one of her flock, for as Matron she is responsible for my welfare. This was the belief of Florence Nightingale, who revolutionised nursing. The doyenne to all trained nurses who followed in her footsteps concluded that the rigorous regime of nursing training could easily breed indifference or lack of feeling. The Victorians' reverence for motherhood may have influenced her to stress on many occasions that it was essential a matron have a maternal feeling for her nurses, a sensitivity often lacking in the next century.

Matron continues to write, lifting a finger on her left hand to point to a box of thermometers on her desk and I move to select one. Suddenly the realisation of how fed up I am with everything at this time turns into anger. There must be some other career path I can follow, with sane hours and less physicality. My tongue takes over, mouthing words that I vaguely know are forming in my head.

'I wish to hand in my resignation, Matron.'

Here is my escape from intimidating pressure, aching weariness, early rising and the regimentation, nothing at all to do with the petty rule associated with a broken thermometer.

At last, recognition. Matron places her pen on the blotting paper pad and studies my face over her gold-rimmed glasses.

'Have you thought this through carefully Nurse? You have been doing very well during the year.'

She still hasn't addressed me by name so how would she know the year has passed satisfactorily? As though standing behind an ecclesiastic lectern all I can say is: 'I may have chosen the wrong path.' Struggling to prevent the tears building, I am angry with myself for showing a lack of control.

The stark white veil surrounding her immobile expression, the frost-coloured complexion, her slim body encased in white partly hidden behind the ponderous desk, Matron might have been a painted portrait, placed beneath the others in a room scantily lit by natural light entering the narrow windows. Her pale fragility is deceiving. Her strength must come from within, she is known by all trainees to have been tested during the First World War while nursing wounded Australian troops in the fierce heat of the Egyptian desert. One of the deprivations was a personal allotment of water, no more than one bucket a day for body cleansing and clothes washing. I doubt whether she would have stood in the sizzling desert sands and cried because she wanted out. She had survived more than I probably would ever be expected to and was one of the army nursing sisters awarded the Florence Nightingale Medal.

'Sit down, Nurse MacSkimming,' is an order and I am grateful to feel the weight lift from my legs, but an increasing headache is pounding against my skull as though, like me, trying to find an escape route out of a tight corner.

10

Back on Course

Two strong women whose reasoning and experience outshine mine are bound to win me over. They are deft at spelling out the advantages of withdrawing my sudden resignation and continuing to strive towards the ever-distant light at the end of the tunnel. This is initiated by clever action on Matron's part in telephoning my mother on the spot, explaining the situation and at the same time I hear her giving some praise of myself and my suitability for nursing. I could have pointed out that I have learned more about cleaning in the past year than nursing. Matron passes the receiver and my mother, ever sensible and diplomatic, suggests I try for a little longer and emphasises the lack of opportunity in a country town. Did I really want to return to work as jack-of-all-trades in the local service station as bookkeeper, clerk and petrol pump attendant? That was the only work available to me at the end of school. Besides, my first year holidays are due.

My impulsiveness may have gained me something. My instant holiday application for four weeks' annual leave is approved and will coincide with my birthday and Christmas.

In the meantime Hygiene lectures take place. These include three pages on the obvious dozen requirements of personal care under the heading The Art of Healthy Living. One essential is a daily hour of exercise spent outdoors in fresh air.

'I've prepared myself just for that, at least for today,' Betty whispers behind her raised hand. We are seated together in the Maitland Lecture Theatre on a warm afternoon. The subject and the enclosed atmosphere make it necessary to fight a persistent drowsiness.

'I've been invited to join in a few sets of tennis with some RMOs later this afternoon,' she explains, fulfilling one essential rule with regard to good health while breaking another, in the forbidden social intercourse with medical staff.

Another inclusion in healthy living standards is eight hours' sleep each night, which makes everyone burst into laughter.

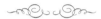

A whole 28 days spent away during the best time of the year to relax in an unspoiled coastal village arrive at last. My parents will be able to repay some of the Burstal family's kind hospitality to me when Janet comes to stay during the last week, arriving on a day that does the area justice. The small town is cradled between the blue coastal range and a rugged coastline of black cliffs linked by miles of golden sand. Town Beach is a short walk from the house where we spend long hours in the warm surf, dunk our sunburnt bodies in cool rockpools and photograph each other posing on the sand. The town's main street is devoid of the boutiques and coffee shops we frequent in the city, but shopping is in our blood so we inspect the stock in the various small departments of Reed's Country Corner Store and must be content with a milkshake in the Niagara Cafe, one of two Greek cafes. At the end of the week the expectation of returning to the city by air is a unique experience, awaited with excitement. Two local residents, the entrepreneurial Dulhunty brothers, have inaugurated an air service between Sydney and Port Macquarie. They are also real estate agents and envisage the fishing hamlet

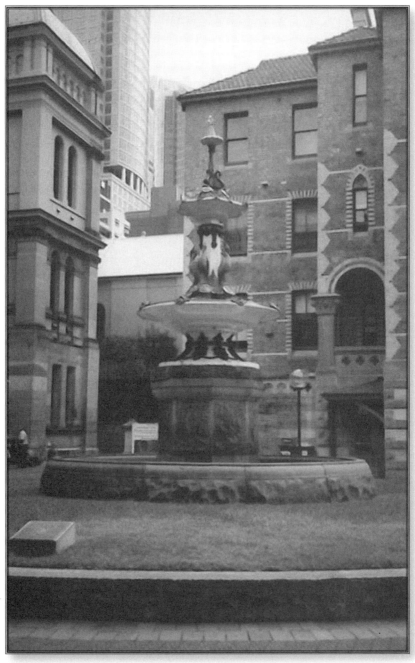

The Robert Brough Fountain (1907) and the Nightingale Wing (1867) in the background are listed on the National Trust Register along with the Sydney Hospital sandstone buildings (1894) that face Macquarie Street.
(Author photograph)

becoming a tourist attraction.

There is no time to feel dejected, as I usually do when saying goodbye to the family. We wave farewell to them standing at the pier's end and enter the flying boat cabin. Following the smiling air hostess's directions we settle into our seats. Janet, with her ambition of joining these ranks, watches her movements with great interest.

The engines turn over and race to pick up speed until the roar of increasing power pulls us out into midstream. The Sunderland's bulbous body gathers speed, splicing the glassy surface of the Hastings River, and through the cabin window we watch the waves surge away from the plane's belly and spread shorewards, washing vigorously among the bordering mangroves. Lifting steadily, then banking towards the south, our course is set to follow the blue Pacific on the left. The Norfolk Island Pines parading in miniature along the town's headland fall behind. In just over an hour we touch down on Sydney Harbour. The engines' roar easing, the aircraft moves gently towards Rose Bay inlet. What could be more convenient? We walk the distance from the landing stage to Janet's home beside the Royal Sydney Golf Course.

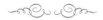

A bundle tied with white tape constitutes my weekly supply of uniforms, marked by name and ready for collection from the laundry at the rear of the Nightingale Wing. The count is rarely correct, something is always missing, which with luck will surface at a later date. Our probationers' caps have been passed in and we graduate to second-year head covering. The difference is the elimination of the side peaks, which are replaced by a straight plain band around the crown and buttoned behind at the base of the hairline.

Following the courtyard path to return to my room, the bundle of fresh linen is tucked beneath my arm. The movement of staff makes a pleasant scene, especially at changeover time as staff criss-cross the green heart of the hospital complex, passing the fountain that I now know to be the Robert Brough Memorial Fountain. Having been absent for four weeks, and perhaps with a freshened outlook, I appreciate the significant activity: sisters in blue, white veils lifting in the breeze, trainees smart in aprons and caps, lots of starch giving body to the garments. Somewhere production in starch factories must be at its highest level. My outlook has changed and I feel a twinge of pride in belonging to the scene, a busy thriving centre for healing the sick in a perfect position to serve a bustling metropolis.

The Annual Report for the year of my commencement, 1949, and which I had leafed through because a copy happened to be on Sister's desk, verified the hospital's important role. The total number of admissions for that year, no doubt similar for this year, for we are already into 1951, is 8,011. Casualty treated over 67,000 and Outpatients 35,000. The number of beds available, excluding veranda beds, was 290, which were attended by 104 Honorary Medical Officers. Veranda beds numbered approximately five per veranda and were positioned on the side of some wards overlooking the inner hospital grounds. Placed parallel to the wall these extra beds are often used to accommodate infectious patients, who have been diagnosed with pulmonary tuberculosis and require barrier nursing: their crockery is kept separate; and a mask, gown and gloves are kept at the bedside and worn when attending their needs; and extra care is taken when emptying their blood-stained sputum mugs. The open veranda fenced in above the stone parapet with wire netting allows complete entry of fresh air, vital for the long tedious healing of their diseased lungs.

An urgent 'Nurse! Nurse!' shouted by a veranda patient gave rise to June's first experience of an emergency. She was just a few weeks out of Tutor School and had been left in charge of the ward. Sister was on a day off and the Senior Nurse was on an evening meal break. Hurrying out to the veranda she found what she later described as imagining how a crime scene might appear when just discovered. A mentally disadvantaged patient in his teens, who had been diagnosed with tuberculosis, was seated on the floor beside his bed playing in a pool of blood. A fit of violent coughing had preceded a severe haemoptysis (coughing up of blood). To keep her moving on with the telling of her story, in unison we expel an appropriate expression of disgust.

'There was blood everywhere,' describing her discovery. 'Spattered up the wall, all over the bedclothes and himself, and the smell, I'll never forget the smell—it was horrible. I ran to the phone in the foyer and paged Medical Boards—what a peculiar expression that is. However, it produced the Medical Registrar very quickly.'

June is pragmatic and never one to be flustered, so we picture her swiftly carrying out the necessary actions in the correct order: supplying gown and gloves for the doctor and following his instructions; fetching a bowl of ice cubes for the boy to suck; then cleaning up, while reassuring the remaining men housed on the veranda, looking on in awe from the security of their beds.

II

I Know Where I'm Going

13 January 1951

Complimentary tickets to attend certain performances of the Borovansky Ballet at the Theatre Royal in Castlereagh Street, occasionally offered to the nursing staff, are very welcome and when available quickly snatched up by several in our group.

Today there is an invitation of another kind pinned to the noticeboard. If accepted this means we will be demonstrating our own dancing skills instead of sitting and watching others perform theirs on stage—provided I can find a partner and not be given the wallflower's role.

Ballroom dancing, learned at country balls and an essential skill, is one of my favourite pastimes,. When presented as a debutante, I circled the Memorial Hall dance floor partnered in the arms of my country farmer.

The host tonight is the Merchant Marine Officers' Club at a venue close by in Phillip Street. Janet, Barbara and I decide to accept. This outing could be an adventure and offer a chance to meet a group of men more than likely from overseas countries and hopefully experienced dancers.

Hooking my newly purchased Dyomee bra at the back, I face the mirror. What a shame it cannot be worn on the outside and seen for its beauty and the work of art it is: on each pink satin cup a middle beginning of machine stitching circles round and round from the centre outwards creating the perfect uplift and the right bodyline beneath my pale blue linen frock with collar and cuffs trimmed in white embroidery. A single strand of graduated pearls, my only necklace, is placed around my throat. Nylon stockings, eased on for the first time, have been stored among my underwear for several years. They had arrived by post in two envelopes, one stocking in each, a gift from Lyle, my old boyfriend serving in the navy. I had been delighted with this entirely new and scarce fabric: the stockings, when pulled up out of the envelope, were engagingly sheer. They prove to be as cloyingly hot as my on-duty thick ones. An extra splash of Evening in Paris perfume tilted out of the dark blue bottle and applied at the base of the neck trickles down into the Dyomee bra depths, giving a final touch.

The golden light of summer's long evening is rapidly fading as we stroll down Martin Place. The sun is dipping behind the city's tallest structure, the AWA Tower, and the incoming night is sultry and humid. Roads are defined by lines of pooled light simultaneously turning on. Neon lights flicker briefly, then off for a few seconds before their vivid colours are set to burn steadily. Turning left into Phillip Street and reaching the given address, we ride the lift up to the top floor. The doors glide open and we are greeted by the mellow notes of a saxophone. Stepping out into a function room with chairs lining the walls, the parquetry floor shines beneath a line of frosted glass light shades. The saxophonist is warming up on a podium at the far end and we take possession of seats placed on the right hand side. The piano player takes the initiative, joins his fellow musician, and a popular melody flows. The first movement of one male crossing the floor sets up a chain reaction of others who follow, choosing a partner, and the floor's lustre quickly disappears beneath moving feet.

A young man wearing a tweed jacket more suitable for northern climes moves swiftly. He is drawing nearer and I hope it is not obvious that I have seen him approaching so I turn my head away. I hold my breath and hope I am not mistaken in the direction he is taking. He holds out his hand and smiles—I am his choice as partner in the first dance. Moving towards the dance floor, my first impressions are of a fair-haired, stockily built person, and as the dance progresses I see his eyes are blue like the summer ocean he sailed in on that very morning. As our conversation progresses I realise his voice is enhanced by a Scottish accent.

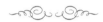

27 January 1951

I hover in the doorway leading out onto the veranda of Ward 15, hoping for a sighting of SS *Hector* sailing towards the Heads. Due to cast off at 12 midday, she should be passing Mrs Macquarie's Chair about now, but there is no sign of her and I can feel Sister's eyes on me. Finally losing her patience she crossly instructs me to keep my mind on the task in hand. This is at the end of two exciting weeks that have brought the Third Engineer aboard SS *Hector*, William Gordon Sim, into my life. The days sped by like a whirling top, until the spin came to an abrupt end with the ship's departure. The past two weeks have been a juggling of his on-duty shifts to fit in with mine so that off-duty time spent together means experiencing some of the entertainment the city has to offer.

Bondi Beach, a generous width of yellow sand lying in a perfect curve on the rim of a vivid blue Pacific Ocean, is packed with sun-seekers. William and I step into the warm ocean, intense

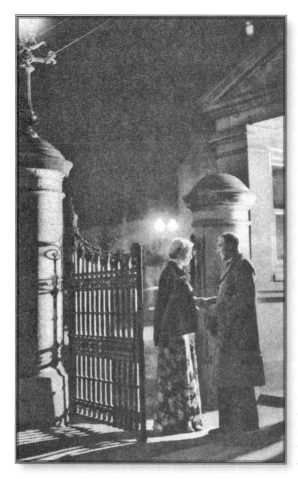

*Saying 'Goodnight' at the entrance to Sydney Hospital. (*Pix *magazine, courtesy of Mitchell Library, State Library of NSW)*

afternoon light, white-capped water rolling in and the thunder of sea green bursting around our bodies as the waves break.

Leaving the water and stretching out on my beach towel, then rolling over, I watch William revelling in the tepid surf, swimming in a line of surfers on the cusp of the furthest breaker. He is a strong swimmer, having learned in the bracing North Sea as a top member of his swimming club. His home town is Fraserburgh, north of Aberdeen on the furthest north-east tip of Scotland, one of many tiny fishing towns that are the backbone of the great herring industry.

'I saw you entering the room the night we met and I kept my eye on you, determined that no-one else would reach you before

I did,' is William's compliment on that first outing.

Some of these times together are spent simply, revealing our different backgrounds, while walking in the city or between boarding fun rides at Luna Park. Wanting to dance together again, we make up a foursome with Barbara and Johnny, William's engineering associate, to dine and dance downstairs at Chequers Nightclub.

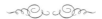

As I step down from the tram William is waiting, beaming with pleasure and he takes my arm reassuringly; this is my first sighting of him in uniform, the whiteness of shirt, trousers and shoes vibrantly spotless. Leaving the Miller's Point tram terminal we follow the road as it curves down to the line of finger wharves in Hickson Road.

I suddenly feel shy, though my reservation does not escape him when much later he reveals his thoughts on that walk down to the harbour—that he'd be daft not to take things easily and coast along like a fair-weather ship. He was afraid he would lose me when we had just met.

The *Hector* is tied up at No. 8 Walsh Bay, looking splendid in the late afternoon sun. Up the gangway and along the deck we reach his cabin amidships, where he will entertain me for the evening catered for by an attentive steward supplying food and drinks in the near new, shipshape Third Engineer's cabin. This is one of Alfred Holt's finest 'sea boats' of the Blue Funnel Line, built in Belfast the previous year, an 18-knot cargo ship carrying a dozen passengers.

A radio is playing softly on the desk and a soulful voice croons 'Bewitched', the latest Rodgers and Hart hit. The sound of laughter and conversation wafts through the open cabin door, indicating someone else is entertaining aboard that night.

The door to the Nightingale Wing will be locked dead on

11 p.m. and I don't have a late pass. I'm reluctant to leave so I suggest overstaying the curfew and entering later by climbing through the ground floor kitchen window, which is never locked. This must be carried out with caution, taking care not to step into the mammoth saucepan of porridge soaking for breakfast. William is quick to shake his head. He doesn't want me to risk being grounded, suggests I stick by the rules and he will arrange for a taxi to take me home. A gentle kiss and he is steering me towards the cabin door. I am unaware, at that stage, of the plan forming in his mind.

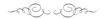

His last remaining night in port has arrived. Aboard a Manly ferry we are entertained on the crossing by the music trio who constantly make the crossing playing piano, violin and accordion for a few pence dropped into their collection box. As we alight, the distant skirling of bagpipes can be heard moving along The Corso. We follow like children at a parade, chasing the haunting pipes and beating drums. The players disband where The Corso meets the ocean and the bordering pines along the Esplanade. A smoky glass sea forms a backdrop beyond the tree trunks.

We sit in silence looking over the smooth ocean, listening to the nor'easter soughing in the pine needles overhead as twilight drops. With the disappearance of the pipe band I feel a sadness and William is quiet, until suddenly there is an outpouring of words. Earnest and loving, he reveals his plans. On his return to Liverpool he will resign, apply to emigrate and join the shifting population of thousands moving 'down under'. Still young at 27, he has no family ties: his parents have passed away and there are no siblings. How did I feel about this? Then a proposal of marriage. Momentarily lost for words I can't answer yes or no but I am positive in my promise to wait.

12

Surreal Nights

Ward 7 is part of the original hospital, a ward for the treatment of men diagnosed with urological problems. There are usually 14 to 16 patients, supervised from a central desk set out in the usual Nightingale format. The placement of the supper room for night staff within the ward's day room lessens the loneliness of my second year night duty. The faint awareness of nurses coming and going, cooking their choice of eggs, chops, bacon and toast, is reassuring. Murmuring voices around the supper table help to make it most unlikely that a prowler may be lurking outside on the faintly lit veranda. Shifty individuals are known at times to rove menacingly around the hospital precincts, to steal or fantasise about the young nurse seen through a ward window. Another reason they may shun this area is that Ward 7's veranda is part of the main thoroughfare for staff moving from the front wards to those at the rear.

An almost cheerful attitude is felt towards going on night duty again. William has telephoned from Melbourne, one of the *Hector*'s homeward-bound ports of call, and several delightful letters full of feeling have arrived along with a studio portrait taken during his Melbourne stay. His continuing correspondence is something I will eagerly await.

Admissions settled in, with fasting signs hung on bedheads, water jugs removed from lockers, sleeping pills handed out before I come on duty, the night hours might not be too labour intensive. The requirements of pre-op enema and pubic shave attended to during the evening by one of the wardsmen, the dark ward is hushed. There is little disturbance, except for a stertorous snort or the padding of slippers as someone heads toward the bathroom at frequent intervals until introduced to the bedside convenience of a male urinal. After all that is why most are here, for open surgery to remove the complete prostate gland or the closed method via the urethra, a trans-urethral resection, resulting in return of a normal urine flow. A reprieve also for those irritable wives disturbed at night by bedclothes flung back across their side of the bed preceding the husband's umpteenth dash to the toilet.

Post-operation night is a different matter. A glass Winchester bottle is hooked onto the bedframe storing the bladder drainage from a rubber catheter and adjoining tubing, the flow moving sluggishly or blocking at times. Blood transfusions in glass flasks, hanging on drip stands and feeding into an arm, must be changed not by nursing staff but by the RMO assigned to each ward. Most catheters flow reasonably. Some are stubbornly reluctant, clogged with viscous debris and blood, a substance that clots or spills, stains or drips onto the floor, sealing floorboard cracks and keeping the nurse constantly running with bucket and mop or filling the laundry trolley with soiled sheets.

Irrigating at the patient's bedside, I gently push the saline out of the purpose built syringe into the catheter and watch hopefully for the fluid's return into the kidney tray; then the ritual is repeated until the returning liquid is clear. The beat of my pounding heart quickens, partly with exertion or a sense of urgency to keep the rubber tubing draining. I try not to make too much clatter in the treatment room during rinsing and re-sterilising equipment and resetting trays ready for the next round of flushing out bloody catheters. Occasionally glass catheters are used in female wards to relieve urinary retention. Avoiding their use, preferring the rubber version, eliminates the horror of glass snapping with a patient's sudden movement.

If time allowed I might have paused and wondered why I have chosen to be here—a ghostly figure, robed in white gown, gloves and mask, moving stealthily throughout this bizarre scene until reason and Mr Richards make it quite clear. Mr Richards' eyes glow in the torchlight watching nervously as the procedure is repeated over and over. His drainage is the most stubborn and I work painstakingly to make it flow again. His body is trembling, whether shivering in fright as I wield the large-scale metal syringe or maybe his body temperature is falling. A hot blanket snatched out of the hot cupboard is a wondrous aid: laid on his upper body it corrects his tremor.

In less frantic times a hot blanket placed around the shoulders of a cold night nurse seated at a lonely desk can revive warmth and her sinking enthusiasm for night duty.

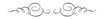

Fated to have a lengthy association with Ward 7, I am delegated to return there at the end of night duty. I don't mind as I know the routine so well and like working in a male ward, especially with the older men, who are mostly easy to get along with and appreciative of the attention they get.

Absorbed in the task at hand, cleaning and rinsing the sludge through used catheters and tubing in preparation for re-sterilisation, my thoughts are elsewhere. More pleasant thoughts than those associated with this chore crowd my mind, now that I have reason to dream and dwell on the future. Sister's voice breaks the spell.

'There is someone asking to see you. He is waiting in the foyer.'

The faint smile on her face indicates this could be something pleasant and I immediately drop what I am doing, wash my hands and hurry to the door. My visitor is standing in the foyer beneath the paging board, various numbers flashing on grey glass above his head. Mr Richards, my friend of the night, is waiting, looking a little uncertain until I appear in the doorway; the deep gutter lines etched into his face and around his mouth relax into a wide smile. He looks a different man out of pyjamas, dressed in well-worn trousers and sports jacket, thick black hair slicked back under a layer of Brylcreem, the daylight heightens the swarthiness of his skin.

'Hello, Nurse,' extending his right arm and a warm handshake.

'You must be wondering how I knew you would still be here—well I checked with Matron's office.' The brown paper bag clutched in his other hand is thrust forward.

'I appreciate what you did for me the night of my operation, a nasty job for anyone to do. You were an angel and I'll not forget it. I've made something for you. A hobby of mine.'

Excitedly, I open then peer into the large bag and pull out his present: a superbly crafted handmade wooden box in walnut, its highly varnished lid is lifted by a knob made from a half cotton reel. I might plant a kiss on his leathery cheek but shyness holds me back, preventing me from expressing my feelings in such a way. As I watch his back disappearing down the stairs I regret not having done so. He has travelled a long distance from the outer suburbs to deliver his special gift to me, his angel of the night. A pleasing compliment given, however difficult to uphold.

Now well into my second year I am more settled with the expectation of an air mail envelope edged in blue and red, waiting in the mail box. Checking each day, then the delight of ripping open the wrapper and an increasing pleasure upon reading through the many pale blue featherweight pages from William.

Surreal Nights 145

His letters are written every Sunday night without fail from his home in Fraserburgh and are filled with news and items that allow me to know him better and I respond in kind. Plans for the future are underway following his arrival back in Liverpool and resignation from the Blue Funnel Line. His application to emigrate is lodged, but the waiting is tedious.

13

The Virgins' Retreat

The Young Street Sydney Hospital Nurses' Annexe comprises four large Victorian terraces on the corner of Young and Bridge streets. The interior has been remodelled so that there is accessibility from one terrace to the next throughout and the houses are similar to a large two-storey house. Two Home Sisters enforce the rules and supervise the functioning of services, which are few. These include overseeing the maid's cleaning and setting up the afternoon and morning tea traymobiles for the Nurses' and Sisters' lounge rooms. A strict eye is kept on discipline, such as the usual 11 p.m. locking of the front door. Sister Galway is severe and dour; Sister Campbell her opposite, sweet and soft. Both have weathered gruelling service, as Matron Pidgeon had in the Egyptian desert, during the First World War. Most of my friends are housed here, quarters teasingly referred to as the Virgins' Retreat. It may be an apt name, as the law-abiding girls domiciled here seem to be as quiet as the atmosphere dominating the hallways and rooms. The social life of those sent down to live in the Eye Hospital day quarters seems to be much busier and more varied than ours.

Barbara and I share a sparsely furnished double room with the usual drab features, although I have scored a commodious

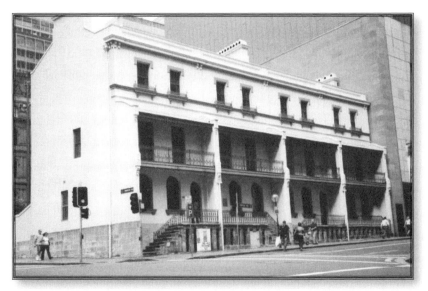

Young Street Nurses' Annexe, 2008, now used as offices. (Author photograph)

dressing table with mirror attached and a separate wardrobe instead of the pokey combination dressing table–wardrobe. Two precious items are placed on top: William's photo portrait and Mr Richards' walnut box, ideal for storing William's letters. The single window looks out over the site of the First Government House. Living conditions are archaic and Spartan; apart from morning and afternoon tea, no meals are supplied. Main meals are to be taken in the dining room of the Nightingale Wing. It's a long walk to breakfast when waking hungry on a day off or when a late shift is scheduled, so we do without and wait until morning tea. A thoughtless arrangement, too. when we are tired after a 6.00 a.m. to 2.00 p.m. shift and have to change and walk back up Macquarie Street for dinner. Board and lodging are deducted from pay and the country girls think at the very least tea, toast and jam might be set out for breakfast on a self-help basis; no butter of course, just as there is bread and jam only to accompany the tea available in the Nightingale Wing before a 6.00 a.m. start.

Walking to and from the hospital in uniform is not allowed but we do anyway in daylight hours, when we decide not to wait for the

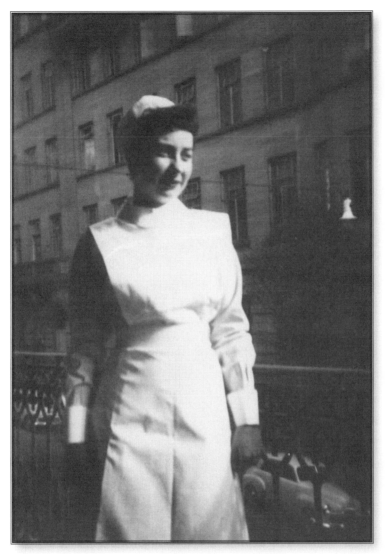

Author standing on the veranda of the Young Street Nurses' Annexe, 1951. (Author photograph)

hospital car or if we have missed it—the walk is often pleasant. Macquarie Street is reached by taking a short cut through Phillip Lane, leading out onto a pavement bustling with doctors hurrying to their rooms, their visiting patients, wigged lawyers and Queen's Counsels and, at certain times, uniformed nurses, resulting in a hub of professional activity.

The public often recognise us with a smile or a man salutes by tipping his hat on passing. We are pleased to be acknowledged as noteworthy and as emphasised in our Tutor School notes, we take pride in our uniform. Walking towards duty we display the brightness of a freshly starched white apron and cap, the no-nonsense comfort of black stockings and low-heeled shoes. Later, off duty and returning towards the Harbour, we are not always spick and span models of propriety, but have rebellious hair loosened around the cap, tired faces and aprons stained during a frantic morning.

The symbols of Nightingale nursing are still apparent, the white aprons indicating that nursing is also domestic and womanly work. The Sisters in Lucy Osburn's day wore neat half aprons and Lucy Osburn's higher authority was emphasised by a lack of apron; the adornment of an ornate cross against her black dress was a corroboration of her position as a Christian and educated lady.

14

A Grim Revelation

The Chapel of St Luke the Physician leading off Ward I is dimly lit, cool in summer, freezing in winter as most places of worship seem to be. It is a sanctuary for those who like to come and pray, whether staff, visitors or patients, and where church services for all denominations are held. The chapel's interior contains original gas fittings, etched glass doors, stained glass windows and, behind the altar, an outstanding tiled mural. Occasionally the venue is chosen by a nurse for the celebration of her wedding at the completion of her training, when marriage is no longer forbidden and a sudden sentiment for years domiciled within these grounds makes the sanctified area her choice.

This rear building, a harmonious design by architect John Kirkpatrick, contains the Chapel and Ward I, and the Worral Theatre on the floor above, with a small room set aside as the RMO's sick bay. Facing east, this picturesque section is unfortunately hemmed in at the rear by the Travers Building, disguising to some degree its architectural symmetry, the corner turrets and the balconies with cast iron lace and columns.

Ward I, the dermatology ward, runs parallel to the Chapel and is a subdued place, not the usual area of frantic activity as other wards can be, unless something unexpected occurs. It is also a smaller ward, providing male and female sections for the care of skin diseases, and treating some who suffer torturous and debilitating afflictions.

Sister Mortimer is the Charge Sister, with a quiet disposition and sometimes, depending on the situation, one that verges on the nervous, who earnestly supervises, with never a raised voice to suit the prevailing atmosphere. The previous week this calm area was stirred into activity by a patient's undiagnosed pregnancy swiftly becoming labour and delivery of a full-term baby out of the rolls of fat which had helped hide her condition. This was followed by the transfer of mother and baby to appropriate care at Crown Street Women's Hospital.

The dermatology ward, always referred to as the 'skin' ward, is a true euphemism and skin the operative word for this strangely inhuman place as humans, unlike some other animals, are not commonly thought of as shedding copious amounts of dried skin flakes. Here they thickly layer the sheets or escape to drift in the air like dust motes suspended in a shaft of sunlight. Shaken out of pyjama legs by the movement of mobile patients, a film is cast over the floor. If the body is slathered with unguents and lotions the oiliness infiltrates gauze bandages, and stains pyjamas, white hospital gowns and freshly changed bed linen. Psoriasis, dermatitis, the rash of secondary stage syphilis, burrowing insects known as scabies, fungal infections and other torments sent to harass the human body are miseries staff endeavour to ease or cure with a strict regime of prescribed treatments. Lukewarm sodium bicarbonate baths are run or poultices created. Cooled starch is spread with a spatula onto a calico square like icing a cake, then a layer of gauze; with the turned in edges of calico holding it together, the gauze side is placed over the weeping area and bandaged in place.

My first set task following breakfast, as the second-year nurse on duty, is taking the used hypodermic needles to be sharpened and made ready for reuse. Situated on the floor above in a room adjacent to the Worral Theatre, the 'instrument' men do this work. Responsible for many tasks, the primary one is setting up and sterilising trays with the appropriate instruments each surgeon requires for an operation, followed by cleaning and storing these after operations. A member of this group attends to the nurses queuing at the doorway, kidney dishes in hand. Standing before a motor driven wheel, dressed in neat white trousers and hospital gown, the instrument man is carefully honing each needle point on the spinning abrasive surface. Occasionally he discards one, weathered by too many sharpenings.

This short break away from the ward might be welcome if there weren't so many treatments waiting to be carried out. As the most senior nurse on duty this morning I hurry back down the stairs and into the treatment room, place the dish of needles into the instrument steriliser and turn the steam tap on. The morning hours quickly pass; Sister has gone to lunch. Mr Kelly is the last on my treatment list, his dressing previously taken down before the night staff went off duty.

The main dressing trolley, a cumbersome metal affair resting on heavy, sluggish wheels, like most hospital furniture, is swabbed down with disinfectant and set up before breakfast. Bottles of solutions fill the bottom shelf. Canisters graduated in size like kitchen canisters are in a row arranged along the top shelf, filled with cloth dressing towels, pads, gauze swabs, cotton balls and bandages, transferred with sterile forceps from metal drums sterilised within the hissing barrel body of an autoclave housed in operating theatre anterooms. The treatment room steriliser has been emptied and refilled with a 2 per cent soda solution; rubber gloves have been rinsed, dried and paired, then boiled for five minutes in a special glove bag placed in a plain water glove steriliser.

Gowned and masked, I push the hefty trolley down the corridor towards the men's end of the ward, loaded with equipment as sterile as any examining bacteriologist might hope for. Keeping in mind the all-important goal of economy, all utensils and linen are washed, re-sterilised and reused.

Mr Kelly's raw open wound, like any other, requires great care to ensure unwanted infection is not introduced. He is sitting upright, his bed placed in a dark corner behind the entrance door into the small ward.

'How are you feeling today Mr Kelly?' I ask in my most cheerful tones hoping for a reply but there is none. The other men in the ward have given up trying to coax a word from him or cheer him up as he sits all day in his flannelette pyjamas, hidden in his dim corner mostly with eyes closed or staring at the back of the door, dealing with his photophobia and his depressed state.

Carefully unwinding circles of offensive, stained bandages, until the last one is loosened and removed, there is still no reaction or emotion shown by Mr Kelly. I know what to expect with the unveiling of the many layered bandages and gauze pads that cover the crown of his head; there is no hair or covering of skin, but a scalp disfigured by furrowed, raw, suppurating flesh.

'Hold still Mr Kelly, I will be as quick as I can.' I try with soothing words to dispel any apprehension he might feel but doesn't reveal now, or at any time. I have promised swiftness, which is out of the question while moistening then lifting pads or Vaseline gauze squares laid across his crown, in case they have become cemented into the open flesh. A corner loosened I gently lift the dressing. Were my eyes playing tricks? Did I see a slight movement beneath the dressing and then I gasp as the area is further exposed to reveal a writhing mass of maggots feeding on the man's flesh. An insect that arouses disgust in everyone, it is imperative I don't reveal this finding to the patient or show my feeling of revulsion. Removing the last pad, disturbing the creatures, wriggling, turning over, their struggle horrible to behold as they wallow in the sloughy wound, I smartly drape a dressing towel over his head and hurry to the phone. I take care not to run, only allowed in the case of fire or emergency, and this problem doesn't fit into either category. The switchboard dialled, the resident doctor assigned to the ward is paged. When Dr Col Jennings promptly appears, his familiar face above the pristine white drill jacket is a welcome sight as he strides into the ward. His arrival means my problem is now shared. I have remained at Mr Kelly's bedside, not sure whether to begin picking out the horrible evidence with dressing forceps. There is a sympathetic expression on the doctor's face and he places a reassuring pat on my shoulder. Later, after his examination, we move out to the treatment room.

'This is not a bad thing, a nasty shock for you and unpleasant for the patient if he learns about it but we may be able to avoid that,' and continuing before settling down at the desk to write in the patient's notes. 'Maggots have been known in past instances, such as infesting war wounds on the battlefield, to clean out the dead tissue—much the same principle as the application of leeches to relieve congested tissue. More effective than a weak solution of Eusol, eh Nurse?' Watching his face closely I wait for some blame. None is given as the sparse hairs of a fledgling moustache part and his lips stretch sideways into a grin.

'Fine,' relieved, turning up my nose. 'I know it's spring and blowflies are plentiful but I wish it hadn't been me who made the discovery.' Feeling more relaxed, I add, 'It's a very different situation when placed purposefully in a wound.'

I am not confident about Sister Mortimer's reaction on her return from lunch. She will probably place responsibility on my shoulders for the actions of the blowfly, which flew in unnoticed with the opening of a door.

In the meantime the RMO and I share the treatment of the wound, he removing the larvae one by one and I cleansing and redressing the wound.

'This is your fault Nurse,' Sister's dark eyes are surveying me with criticism. Judged unfairly I dare to speak up, pointing out that flyscreens are non-existent, the wound so tender that firm bandages cannot be applied and there is every chance this occurred before I came on duty. A sideways glance and her eyes narrow.

'Go to lunch, Nurse.'

Rolling down my sleeves and placing my cuffs in position I feel surprised and pleased with myself in speaking out, but have little appetite for lunch. Instead I begin pondering on my time spent as a shopgirl at Curzons and how I attended classes arranged by the management with a view to becoming a fashion buyer. Perhaps I should have persevered with that.

15
Two City Shootings and an Explosion

A wailing ambulance speeding along Macquarie Street, approaching the gates and turning into the hospital grounds, will silence the siren if the patient being transported is not an urgent case. In severe instances, the siren continues to whine until the Casualty entrance is reached and staff hurry to meet the incoming patient.

Ward 1 is in close proximity to Casualty and I am made aware of the arrival of an urgent case as an ambulance makes its noisy transit around the corner of the skin ward. Soon everyone learns what type of injury has been brought in. An admission of someone suffering gunshot wounds is not a common one—one might say it is a most uncommon occurrence.

The shooting occurred in busy Martin Place. A vengeful husband had descended the stairs leading down into a basement shop, aiming at close range and hitting his estranged wife as she stood behind the counter before fleeing up and out of the shop's only entrance. Life-threatening cases such as the Martin Place victim are quickly assessed on arrival then rushed up to Ward 9 and the 'shock bed'. Ideally, the patient is stabilised and then transferred to the operating theatre or, depending on the case, sent directly to theatre. From there the patient is nursed in the relevant ward until recovery or otherwise.

The 'shock bed', first bed to the right of Ward 9's entrance, is always made up in readiness. The top bed linen is folded in the manner of a post-operation bed, allowing easy folding back to the bottom; an intravenous outfit is hung on a metal stand ready to administer saline or blood; as well as an oxygen cylinder, nasal tubes, sucker to the side and bed blocks at the bedhead. The locked 'shock' cupboard on the wall contains trays set up with necessary instruments for examination, inserting a tracheotomy tube or catheter, plus dressings, bandages, splints and medications, including adrenalin that is drawn up and injected straight into the heart muscle if the organ should cease functioning. A sign on the door warns staff against borrowing or lending any article therein.

During attendance on the traumatised patient the four points of care are essentially dispensed as set out in the golden rule of the treatment of shock: Rest, Warmth, Morphia and Fluids.

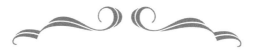

Calamity

Unthinkable—shocking ... *expostulated the horrified citizens of Sydney.*

A royal prince has been shot in their midst on a day that should have been filled with uninterrupted merry-making.

Prince Alfred, Duke of Edinburgh, 24-year-old second son of Queen Victoria and visiting commander of HMS Galatea, has been murderously attacked at a charity picnic, while mingling with his mother's subjects.

Mid-afternoon on 12 March 1868; a peaceful autumn day in Sydney, with the harbour surface flat as a mill pond, HMS Galatea rides serenely at anchorage. The Prince moves through the compressed crowd of picnickers, accompanied by his equerry and an untold number of officials. Some dozen officers and crew from the Galatea add colour to a scene Sydneysiders are sure will never be forgotten.

However the Prince is not followed exclusively by massed devotees of the British crown. As the royal party move across the picnic ground an Irishman, Henry O'Farrell, who is nursing a grudge, pushes in closer. England's refusal to create an independent Irish state is an insult to O'Farrell and the bitterness seethes in his heart. Not placated by the free champagne and beer that flows copiously or a share of the plentiful food that fills the stomachs of the 1,500 or so citizens, O'Farrell is further fired up by the alcohol.

He lifts his pistol, aiming at the Prince whose back is turned to him while observing Indigenous subjects demonstrating one of their dances. The young Prince attempts to clutch his lower back and with a loud groan falls to the ground.

Shouts of 'The Prince has been shot' carry across the grounds, setting off a great panic, some people weeping at this outrage perpetrated in their flourishing colony, outpost of the Empire. Others set upon the gunman with a vengeance. A rope and gibbet is swiftly prepared in a nearby tree and a lynching is imminent until swiftly prevented by the Prince's companions and the police. The wailing set up by those on the outer edge of the crowd continues, for no-one can see clearly whether the Prince is dead or alive.

'Lift him quickly, one person to each leg,' shouts a naval lieutenant from the Galatea. 'But not too rough. Mind you go carefully.'

The Prince's face is ashen with the stricken expression of a wounded man in deep shock.

'Two more lads, one to each shoulder and I'll take care of his head.' The lieutenant keeps a close eye on his subordinates as the men lift the Prince, relieved that someone has taken charge.

As his body rises up, supported by so many hands, a vivid scarlet patch of grass is left behind. Blood is escaping from the wound and is caked on his uniform jacket. Someone grabs a picnic tablecloth and ties it around the Prince's torso. Another order is shouted by the young lieutenant.

'Quickly into the longboat. Someone clear the way.'

Several sailors jump into the Galatea's beached longboat to man the craft, while others help lift the inert body up and over the gunwale. Many willing hands push and pull the wooden vessel away from Clontarf Beach out into deep waters and those rowing put all the muscle power they can muster into their strokes.

Rounding Middle Head, they are urged on by the lieutenant, nursing the Prince's head in his lap. There is a long distance to negotiate, following the width of late afternoon sun glinting like a pathway on the water, until the jetty at Government House is finally reached.

Iron wheel rims turn on flagstones with a reverberating clunk, louder than usual and drummed by the extra speed of a carriage entering the Infirmary grounds. An assistant seated next to the driver jumps down, leaving him holding fast to the reins and quieting his horses with loud instructions. The groom runs towards the hospital entrance seeking out Miss Osburn. She is asked to hasten by return carriage to Government House. Her assistance is needed urgently to organise the nursing of Prince Alfred.

However, Miss Osburn is cautious about her presence being sought without some kind of official approval from Sir Henry Parkes, hesitating before making any decision in attending to the royal personage. This is soon granted and Lucy Osburn hurries from the building out to the waiting carriage, accompanied by Haldane Turiff and Annie Miller, for she has already formed a plan in her mind.

As the carriage enters the gates of Government House, twilight is closing in and a short distance down the grassy knoll the harbour will soon be concealed.

Solitary lights emerge on the northern shore and further to the east, beyond the bushy headlands where Clontarf hides on the rim of the Spit, there is silence. Dust churned up by the hundreds of milling feet trampling the picnic ground earlier in the day, stirred up by the southerly breeze, rises in swirls then settles. A layer of the powdery silt conceals the blood red patch that is a reminder of the day's drama.

Two officials, one each side of Lady Belmore, are waiting at the entrance to Government House. The sudden reining in of the horses, wheels crunching into gravel, sends handfuls flying onto the bordering lawn. A hasty greeting and the three visiting ladies are shown into a stately foyer. Passing an open door on her left, Lucy can see into the visitor's reception room, where a cluster of officials with grim faces stand in a circle waiting for news.

Miss Osburn instructs her companions to wait, and they are shown to seats near the entrance by a silent footman. She alone enters the Prince's apartment and is greeted by the Naval Surgeon. Motioned to move to the side of the four-poster bed she looks down on the Prince's handsome pale features, turned slightly to one side, a bolster placed along his back to keep him in position. He has been changed into a pyjama jacket of the finest cream silk.

How strange, being so new to the Colony herself, that within a week of her arrival she should be standing at a Prince's bedside in charge of his physical comfort.

'Your Highness,' the Surgeon gently addresses his patient. 'This is Miss Osburn, newly arrived from England. She will see to it that competent nurses are available to you.'

The Prince's acknowledgement is a slight nod of his head and the gentle opening then drooping of his eyelids.

The surgeon, a middle-aged man of great dignity and charm, questions Lucy as he takes her by the elbow, directing her to the other side of the room.

'What are your thoughts at this stage on the nursing of the Prince, Miss Osburn? I will be removing the bullet tomorrow morning ... a hair's breadth from his spine and lodged in one rib. Then we can look forward to a great improvement in his condition, I am certain.'

'I will introduce you to the two nurses I have chosen to care for the Prince's well-being. Sister Haldane Turiff will cover the night hours and Sister Annie Miller the daytime. They are both excellent women and efficient nurses.'

'I respect your choices Miss Osburn and I'm sure, as His Highness recovers, he will too.' The surgeon's reply is full of confidence.

Nursing the Prince is a great honour, which can only place the English Sisters in favour with the public and lift the status of nursing in the colony.

Later that evening when Lucy clasps her hands and lowers her head in prayer, she recites a special invocation for the Prince's recovery. She also keeps within her soul a secret thank you for this opportune drama, if it must happen, presenting itself just at the beginning of their time in Australia.

The Prince's service in Her Majesty's Royal Navy has not been one of absolute privilege, but it has kept his health in good stead. A life at sea is a hard one that keeps the seafarer fit, even for a Prince and Commander, so that his constitution is strong and he recovers without any setback.

During this time of healing, Miss Osburn visits Government House twice daily, a short walk from the Infirmary. She is delighted when the Naval Surgeon treats her as a person of his standing and level of intelligence, explaining the medical history and progress of the Prince's recovery.

The Prince invites Lucy to join him at dinner at Government House and, later, to dine aboard the Galatea.

Lucy muses on her situation. How fortunate to be abroad, raw though this country may be, in such elite company.

The Sisters' resentment of Miss Osburn, which had its beginning on boarding the Dunbar Castle when Lucy was allotted a single cabin, is rekindled by these invitations, which are not offered to Haldane or Annie, despite their devoted nursing of His Highness. They are not overlooked however, each receiving the gift of a handsome gold watch and chain from their patient.

The catalyst in these happenings, Henry O'Farrell, having escaped a lynching, languishes in Her Majesty's prison for a time but in the end cannot escape the horror of the noose looped around his neck.

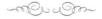

William's letter, as always, is long and full of his hopes for the future and feelings of frustration at not already being on his way back to Australia. Replying in kind, I feel the days are wasted without him being here. Already close to October he has heard nothing positive about his application to the Australian immigration department. In order to earn some income he has taken a position at the Consolidated Pneumatic Tool Company, where he had worked out his apprenticeship before going to sea. He has moved in with his cousin Mary Gordon and her family, packed up his mother's home, watching out every day for the arrival of mail from me and the immigration department.

Re-reading his letter in the Nurses' Sitting Room I do not allow William's frustration to alter my mood of optimism. His determination is stronger than his disappointment, and he adds the news that he is learning to drive, has joined the Freemasons, is keeping fit by rejoining his old swimming club in preparation for his life down under and also putting money aside, something that is impossible for me to do.

On the subject of money William has written more: 'which brings me to the request you made in your letter "to book a passage out and forget the migration scheme". Well Norma you certainly took my breath away and yet when I thought it over I wondered why you had never asked me before. But Darling I can certainly explain why your request is more or less out of the question although I love you more than anything in the world and here is an opportunity to prove it, I can't. I probably could afford to pay the fare out to Sydney but it would leave me flat and I can't leave myself in such a position. I look upon this small amount of money as my only means of being independent and I can't lose that. Am I forgiven?'

Reading his letter quietly with only a few nurses in the room, then reaching the end, I stare moodily out of the window before dropping my eyes and, for the first time, taking a thorough look at the only new addition placed in the room since my arrival. It is a large console, a gift comprising record player, radio and speakers, plus storage, placed against the wall opposite where I am seated: a brass plate secured on the shining veneer is inscribed with an appreciation from a ship's crew for the long, intensive care given by the nursing staff attending their general needs and dressing the horrific burns suffered by injured sailors.

It commemorates the previous 25 January 1950, when the one 'shock' bed in Ward 9 was inadequate. It's a day I remember only by sound, not by being involved owing to my junior status;

the hour when several ambulances followed one after the other, sounding their warning down the full length of driveway and revealing the blackened bodies of barely alive sailors of the Royal Australian Navy.

A fiery explosion on the harbour aboard HMAS *Tarakan* had taken the lives of seven of their shipmates and one dockworker. The men had to be reached by cutting a hole through the ship's hull while others lying injured on deck were being quickly transported to Sydney Hospital. Casualty, alerted, was ready and waiting. Sister Bridgeman with her World War One experience in dealing with numbers of casualties, her long legs speedily conveying her across the courtyard to the Travers Building, had removed her cuffs on arrival, rolled up her sleeves and organised the Casualty area.

The injured sailors are given sedation, followed by the slightly dulled, excruciating misery of dressings soaked and removed and blisters cut. An application of fresh acriflavine gauze or Tullegras is re-applied, made from cotton window netting cut to size and spread with melted Vaseline then packed in flat tins and autoclaved. Later in the progression of healing comes the indulgence of a Lux bath and attempts to prevent scarring skin contractions.

The Nurses' Sitting Room is a stopover, not a place to relax for any length of time, since it is either crowded with staff waiting to go on duty or taking a few minutes' rest during a meal break, or empty so that a long-playing vinyl disc spinning on the turntable is seldom heard, nor does the green radio dial glow with use. It doesn't matter that the console just stands there like a memorial: the sentiment is important, the knowledge that others have been helped in their time of need.

16

Surprises Prompt Contrasting Emotions

'I feel as though I have spent the whole of my life travelling in this train.' I turn restlessly in the carriage seat and gaze out of the window at the dense grey-green bush slipping by. 'Like a nomad continually moving through a desert landscape that hardly alters, only my camel is this government railway carriage.' And indeed I am travelling north once more, but this time the journey will include a stopover along the way.

The response from the opposite window seat is a quick laugh.

'You love going home,' Barbara replies. She is invited to stay with my parents this time and is not complaining. Instead she is enjoying her first trip on the North Coast Express and looking forward to disembarking at Taree before boarding a bus for Forster.

'Of course I do, I just wish I could afford to fly every time.'

In a valiant effort to save I now have £12 in the bank and, in the way of an asset, a bottle of pink champagne, a present from Kay my schoolfriend and companion during our unsuccessful stint as shopgirls. Kay and her new fiancé had taken me out to dinner on my twenty-first birthday. The gift of champagne is carefully wrapped inside my suitcase and I am yet to decide whether I will share it when we join Betty and Elaine for a week's holiday by the sea or keep it for William's return.

Our first impression on arrival is one of slight shock as we drop our cumbersome suitcases at the door to the basic accommodation and greet our friends. We hadn't given much thought to our lodging—we were just pleased to join in with the arrangement.

The rickety, frail-looking stationary caravan sits in an almost deserted caravan park on a headland close to the beach. With a roof curved like a half moon, the squat plywood box has windows large enough to admit the scorching sun but small enough to keep out the cooling north-easterly breeze. Outside is a wobbly card table, balanced on the wooden slabs sunk into the earth and running the caravan's length, where we dine al fresco then wash up in a tin dish. A frame overhead built out of crooked eucalyptus branches is meant to support a canvas covering, which we don't have, so the only shade is underneath a ring of trees on the park's outer edge, several hundred yards away. The sea's close proximity, however, is perfect.

Elaine had begun her training with a previous Tutor School, but had fallen behind and had to make up time when all her sick leave and extra time had been taken becaue of an unfortunate dive into shallow water at Bondi. Luckily she was moved and transported correctly by ambulance to Sydney Hospital, where the diagnosis on X-ray was of a fractured cervical vertebrae. She spent several months in traction, nursed in the Nurses' Sick Bay, but has no qualms about re-entering the surf. Barbara is an avid reader—her legacy of milk-white Irish skin means she mostly, but not entirely, avoids the beach, preferring to spend most of the day reading under shade.

The week is successful although uneventful, and roughing it has turned out to be fun. We are due to leave the following day and spend the last golden afternoon stretched out on the unspoiled beach. Breaking surf and a few solitary seagulls quarrelling over some tasty morsel are vague background sounds in an otherwise peaceful scene, until Betty breaks the spell, standing and shaking the sand from her beach towel. She admits to having a date, the result of a conversation struck up in the main street that morning. We remaining three doze on, the warm tide creeping up over our feet, but still we don't move.

It is not long before curiosity rouses us into a sitting position with the whirr of a small aeroplane engine increasing in sound on approach. The Tiger Moth is moving rapidly in our direction—almost above us, it lifts suddenly and roars past. The wings sway in a salute before disappearing up and over the headland out of sight. We cannot recognise the two leather-encased heads, goggles in place, waving from the cockpits and passing at a meteoric speed. Returning in the dark later that evening, our solitary kerosene lamp glowing in the caravan park to show her the way, Betty confirms our suspicions about the joy-riders' identity.

Our 'snaps' record the week for posterity, photos that portray beach belles in cotton one-piece 'swimmers', shirred with elastic at the back above the waist, and for modesty's sake a skirt stretches over the abdomen from waist to thigh hiding the covering material between the legs. Trendy round lenses framed in white and rubber bathing caps are essential accessories. I attach my latest purchase—white Roman-style sandals with thin straps that wind up and around the calf—which has stalled the addition of another 20 shillings to my bank account. The sandals are an absolute necessity when crossing to the beach as a guard against bindi-eyes in the grass, painful if they spike the tender sole of a foot.

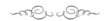

When we return to the hospital, the usual sinking feeling in the pit of my stomach is reduced with the prospect of mail waiting. I can see the distinctive markings of an airmail envelope protruding from the mail box. Sometimes there are small surprises within a packet stamped with a Scottish postmark: tourist booklets recounting the history of Fraserburgh and Aberdeen, containing photos of historical buildings and castles throughout Aberdeenshire; heather pressed between the pages of a letter; or sheet music for the song 'A Gordon for Me', showing William's pride in his second name and his mother's maiden name. Earlier in December a twenty-first birthday present of Robert Burns's poetry, bound in tartan cloth, had arrived.

There are two envelopes addressed to me in the mail box. The first is marked Overseas Cablegram, a rare form of correspondence for me to receive. Holding my breath, I eagerly rip open the envelope.

Monday 31 December 1951

Darling sailing date 30th January see you in April letter following,
   William.

The cablegram has been lying for a week in the pigeonhole. I tear open the letter also dated 31 December.

This afternoon I performed one of the most pleasant duties I have done for ages in sending you a cablegram with my sailing date. The Blue Funnel Line replied to my application to work my way out to Australia and offered me a position as a supernumery engineer on the Diomed. *Unfortunately not one of their new class vessels like the* Hector *and will take quite a few weeks longer to get to Aussie than the four weeks the* Hector *class takes, but I will be on my way to you. I am very pleased not to be a passenger as my work on board won't make the trip feel so long. The only time I want to be a passenger on a ship is when I take you back to Scotland for a holiday. Then I will have you, and you me, and the rest of the ship can do as they please!*

My mind is working like an adding machine trying to calculate everything in terms of work coming up, hoping I will be off night duty by the time he arrives. Maybe he will reach Sydney too late to share with me the four days off at the end of night duty. I must reply as soon as possible with a hastily written aerogram posted at the GPO. There is something I must do first as I hastily turn towards the dining room and run down the stairs hoping to find someone with whom I can share my news.

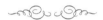

The Fracture Clinic is conducted in Casualty in a room permeated by natural light. This is a pleasant assignment, with normal hours eight to five-thirty, attended by an agreeable, efficient Registrar, John Reimer, and for a few weeks I will assist him. Plaster of Paris, which is inclined to drip or splatter over everything, is at least easy to soak, apply, mould and tidy up when removed from bowls and instruments. It has has a gentle, clean odour, unless blood has soaked into the interior of a plaster cast, creating, a stale smell that is offensive when the cast is cut away with plaster shears.

The clinic is supervised by the Casualty Sister-in-charge, an overseer with a fierce reputation, not so much as a screamer but as one who can be coldly cutting, an opinion expressed by most young nurses. Fortunately for me, after her morning inspection she leaves the Fracture Clinic to function under our capabilities.

The Nurses' Sick Bay is situated on part of the top floor, above

Casualty and the Fracture Clinic, where following a call from Matron's office I have been sent to work out the remainder of my shift.

The doors swing open smoothly, but the inside area is quiet and stuffy, having been closed up for several days or even longer. Everywhere is spotless and tidy, mainly because the beds are empty and made up in laundered perfection. I move around pushing up windows. The day outside is humid and hot, the muggy air is beginning to stir lightly with the arousal of a nor'-easter, wafting in to dispel the stale air.

With the expected admission of a nurse for observation, I set about preparing a room containing one bed, turning the bedclothes down neatly in preparation for her arrival. There is no no need to place a water jug and glass on the locker, as the patient is fasting and I hook the appropriate sign onto the bedhead and make myself familiar with cupboard contents, checking out storage of articles and equipment that might be needed.

This is a novelty, nursing just one patient, and perhaps there will be a chance to sit down now and then in one of the armchairs placed in the four-bedded room near a window. There may also be time to reflect on the harbour, which can be viewed to the north or east from sick bay, spread out like a vast deep blue lake in perfect sunshine.

Upon her arrival I recognise but do not personally know the senior nurse, who is in her last year of training. Smiling reassuringly, I assist the nurse out of the wheelchair, a clumsy affair like all those scattered throughout the hospital departments, which has a wooden seat and arms, and large wheels with metal rim and spokes.

Transferring to the bed, the girl is slow to rise to her feet and reluctant to release her grip on the wheelchair armrests; she is obviously in pain. The motion of suddenly bending forward holding her stomach, breathing in and out in rapid succession coincides with the Assistant Medical Superintendent's arrival. A tall, reticent, fair-haired man, he helps me settle her into bed before swiftly beginning his examination, taking great care over evaluation of the lower abdominal area.

He stands back for a moment contemplating the patient thoughtfully. Meanwhile the nurse's breathing has steadied with an easing of the cramping pain. The small dose of intramuscular pethidine administered in Casualty is beginning to take effect. She manages a feeble smile and, framed by a wealth of curly auburn hair, her pale face accentuates the ginger freckles that dot her nose and cheeks.

Dr Farrar passes on his instructions while writing in the medical notes.

'Appendicitis can't be ruled out. The results of her white cell count may very well be an indication of that. Meanwhile keep a close observation—temperature, pulse and respiration chart recorded half-hourly. Her blood pressure is satisfactory for now and I will reassess that in about half an hour.'

I wonder why the nursing staff are not entrusted with this simple procedure, which would relieve some of the workload placed on medical staff.

'Oh, and put her on a pad check chart,' said over his shoulder as he hurries to the door and a final directive. 'Page me if you are worried about anything.' And the door swings shut behind his disappearing white coat.

With the nursing notes up-to-date and necessary observation charts prepared, I turn to the Superintendent's medical comments to check his findings and a temporary diagnosis of 'abdominal pain due to onset of menstruation'. After checking and recording her blood loss as moderate, this is a possibility.

My patient is restless again, moving from side to side, trying to find a more comfortable position and I stay at the bedside observing carefully, while trying to reassure her with a comforting word.

It becomes necessary to slip out of the room for a few moments to retrieve a vomit bowl just in case, and while at the end of the corridor a wail is set up, a call that might be expected from an animal trapped in the wild. By the time I reach the door of the room her wailing has subsided into a whimper. The patient is sitting up, bedclothes flung back, her startled pallid face looking down between her legs. Reaching the bedside I draw in a sharp breath, followed by, 'Oh, goodness.'

The Senior Nurse reaches out towards me with tears welling up in her eyes.

'Oh God, I'm sorry.'

'It's OK, it's OK,' and I pat her extended arm.

The drawsheet covering the protecting mackintosh that stretches across the width of the bed is saturated, and a tiny lifeless foetus no larger than a minuscule kewpie doll floats in a crimson pool of blood and uterine debris. Swift collection of a metal dish from the pan room as a receptacle for the rolled up drawsheet gathered from beneath the girl, a dash back to the pan room to deposit and keep the specimen for the doctor's inspection, a quick phone call to page him and I am back at the bedside.

Her girlish face glistens with perspiration, which I gently wash, then I sponge her lower torso and legs, and position pads and tuck in fresh linen. When the doctor enters the room the patient is lying with eyes closed, curled up on her side like the recently expelled foetus.

His examination carried out on both patient and the sad evidence, exiting the pan room Dr Farrar lowers his voice as we retrace our steps to the desk. The expression on his face is stern. 'You must on no account relate this to any of your fellow nurses or to anyone for that matter,' he says confidentially, his eyes searching my face.

'Of course not,' and I admire his concern for the patient's feelings and reputation. 'I understand how she must feel.'

However I do not understand why I wasn't warned of the impending outcome and feel some annoyance at not being told of the true diagnosis and the expected ending, which both doctor and patient must have foreseen.

Nothing remains to be discussed, as it is not my place to question the doctor's decision or the motives of any doctor. Perhaps he would have given me more information when due back to check his patient as promised. The doctor's next task is to telephone theatre and arrange a time for the curettage necessary to prevent further heavy bleeding. I wonder if the theatre staff will be sworn to secrecy; the final outcome will be written up in the notes, but will Matron be informed? The answers don't matter. I can't help thinking a problem has been solved for the hapless nurse and, as for me, I will be true to my promise and not reveal to my friends any details of the afternoon's experiences.

Lying in bed that night when sleep escapes the brain and the day's events persist in entering, I am reminded of an excerpt from the Florence Nightingale Pledge for Nurses, read in Tutor School and recited by nurses on Graduation Day.

> *[I] will hold in confidence all personal matters committed to my keeping and all family affairs coming to my knowledge in the practice of my calling.*

Last thought for the day before sleep is captured: Numbers 9 and 10 of the Indispensable Qualities Desirable in a Nurse, Reliability and Obedience, have been encountered and dealt with accordingly.

17

In the Land of Nod and Bedlam

Bethsheba Ghost, what an intriguing name for a pioneer whose story deserves to be told. Her story is, no doubt, a colourful one and her appealing name would suit a main character. An ex-convict and Matron Housekeeper of Sydney Infirmary for 14 years from 1852 to 1866, she had supervised an institution with a grandiose exterior but an interior filled with early Victorian unhygienic practices. She was condemned by some but was dedicated to her position.

Bethsheba, a sophisticated biblical name, and Ghost excites my imagination in the eerie surroundings I find myself in at this moment.

The torch flashes ahead across Ward 4's floor, my slippers muffle my footsteps as I pass on a round of my patients. Right and left the ward verandas enveloped in gloom are a perfect stage for a midnight walk by Bethsheba's ghost. I feel a shiver run through my body although the night is balmy, then my mind rationalises this possibility, reminding me that Bethsheba's mortal habitat had been the original hospital buildings of deplorable construction, demolished in 1881, so that if her ghost wished to revisit surely the replacement buildings would be an unsuitable haunt.

Night duty eventuated this week as hoped for, so I will be finished in early April, coinciding with the *Diomed's* arrival. William's letters, written along the route in his familiar endearing style and posted from Cape Town and Durban, describe a journey of unrelenting work and frustration for the engineers, keeping the ageing ship's engines turning. It is a vessel fit only for the scrap-heap, William wrote, a ship that could be filled with engineers and still things would not go smoothly. In his case, his payment is just one shilling a month! If he can face such a tough journey in order to return to me then it is, in my mind, essential that I deal with stoicism any difficulties I might encounter in the intervening weeks. Lectures on the nursing of medical cases are completed and Ward 4 men's medical ward will bring to life some cases highlighted in Sears *Medicine for Nurses*.

A few patients slumber soundly until jarred awake by a snore reaching its climax and descending once more into oblivion. Quiet by day, others change on the arrival of the night nurses. Some patients have the weakened heart of congestive cardiac failure or narrowed carotid arteries that reduce the flow of oxgen to the brain and cause the patient to become confused. Some with a history of alcohol abuse who are now deprived of drink become obstreperous and suffer the associated hallucinations of the DTs.

The rattling of metal against metal sends a slight warning at first, then grows stronger with increased shaking. Upon inspection, Mr O'Leary's luminous eyes are shining, reflecting the glow of the torch held in my hand. Lying on his side, naked from the waist down, his pyjama trousers have been kicked to the base of the bed amongst the tangled bedclothes. Feeling free of restricting clothing he has defecated into his bed, his bony arms are capable of a surprising strength as he grasps and vigorously shakes the cot sides, calling out for some long lost person in his past.

'Sh, Mr O'Leary, you're waking everyone. Be quiet.'

'Molly,' Mr O'Leary cries. 'Darling Molly give us a kiss darlin'.'

His oxygen mask is lying beside his pillow, torn off in his delirium. This is quickly replaced—perhaps deprivation of oxygen is exacerbating his restlessness and he will settle behind the rubber mask covering his nose and resting on his lips.

'That's not a kiss my luv,' Mr O'Leary laments loudly, pulling the mask off and raising his voice in anger. 'Why don't you do as I ask, girl?'

There is more metallic clattering of cot sides and groans arise from other quarters as patients are wakened. From out of the gloomy depths at the ward's farthest end someone demands he shut up and go back to sleep.

Mr O'Leary is gaining strength, a surprising extra burst from such a frail body he pulls himself into a sitting position then, turning on his knees in his expelled bowel contents, attempts to lift one leg over the railing. Thwarted by withered muscles and giving up on the effort, he falls back onto the pillows. Hanging over the bed rails, speaking all the while trying to placate him, I smartly pull back to avoid his swinging arm. I'm not quite quick enough in side-stepping his hand while he, clutching my cap, takes it into the bed with him; my newly acquired cap with the band shaped into three standing scallops showing that I am now in third year and able to administer injections, one of which is about to be dispensed to Mr O'Leary.

The short pharmacology course I had found interesting—the Latin abbreviations used in prescription writing, understanding where to administer drugs and medicine, when and how much. I carefully read the prescription for Mr O'Leary's sedation, file and snap open the ampoule and draw up the contents. The

In the Land of Nod and Bedlam 177

relieving Senior Night Nurse arrives to check the drug and dosage administered into the upper outer quadrant section of Mr O'Leary's buttock. As the painful solution is eased from the syringe into the tissue he is cursing loudly at Molly's abuse of his person.

Together, the other nurse and I turn, wash and change Mr O'Leary. The smell of paraldehyde, a disagreeable, immediately identifiable odour excreted through his pores hangs like a noxious miasma over his bed. Paraldehyde, an oily substance administered via a wide bore needle, is an amazing sedative insofar as it has the ability to hold back on its effectiveness until dawn is breaking, when the patient, curling up, falls asleep with the arrival of the day staff. There can be several obstreperous patients at one time caged in cot sides and if needed a night wardsman is available. Even more heartening is the presence in the ward of a burly policeman sitting in the darkness at the bedside of an attempted suicide. Suicide is a prosecutable offence, and the offender must be watched until fit enough to be charged. This strong young male presence is welcome. He will assist if necessary in restraining a patient while sedation is made ready, provided he is not too far removed from his prisoner.

There is a certain rapport between the two government bodies, nursing staff and police. Dealing with the general public, the police are often in and out of Casualty and involved with patients. When on day duty a passing paddy wagon is always a certainty for a lift from Young Street to the hospital gates.

Ending my shift in Ward 4, my mode of transport is the hospital car on hand following breakfast to move the night nurses to quarters at Darling Point, a building purchased the year before, 1951, which houses 30 night nurses, the antithesis of Young Street Annexe. Leaning back, my head lying against the headrest in the back seat of the black limousine, I almost doze off, thinking of Janet who resigned as expected and sailed to England with her parents at the end of two years' training. Letters received are full of her news. She has achieved her ambition of becoming an air hostess, being accepted by BOAC after three gruelling interviews, during one of which a member of the panel questioned her ability to name and prepare cocktails for first class passengers. What was her favourite cocktail? To the best of my knowledge Janet has no experience in this area, except for the tasting of a Pimm's No. 1 Cup or a Brandy Crusta. Janet thought quickly, 'A Southerly Buster' she replied. None of the interviewers had heard of this. She had quickly devised her own cocktail.

'How do you mix it?'

Maybe they didn't know either, as 'Southerly Buster' is a name given to a strong Sydney wind. She had invented her own cocktail and her answer must have made an impression for she was accepted. Janet flew in Comets for a short period, but following several crashes, the Comets had been grounded. Thank goodness she was not involved, but one of my letters to her had been. Salvaged from a disastrous crash in Singapore, a mailbag contained the charred letter, with the address still intact and was forwarded on in the tradition of 'the mail must get through'. Janet misses the Comets, writing that the lesser vibration was an improvement on flying in either Skymasters or Constellations. Another one of our original group has resigned. Pauline is to marry her fiancé, who is a pilot in the Royal Australian Navy's Fleet Air Arm. So now we are five.

The hospital car pulls up outside Travencore, a spacious two-storey mansion set in pleasant gardens and quiet surroundings. The interior is carpeted throughout, retaining some of the original antique furnishings, including a piano. The windows look out across Double Bay, easily reached by steps set in the intervening sloping terrain. A sympathetic Home Sister acquires food for afternoon tea that relates to the upmarket surroundings: scones, jam and cream, and a variety of fresh sandwiches and assorted cakes—a cut above the madeira cake and Arnott's Nice biscuits served at Young Street. We wonder why the Young Street Home Sister has not matched these improvements. God bless the Hospital Board of Directors who must be responsible for Travencore's purchase.

A room shared with Elaine, and the luxury of her radio brings pleasure before and after sleep. The small bakelite appliance broadcasts the latest hits, bringing some normality into a turned around sleeping pattern, which is never as refreshing as sleep at night.

It is a pity that most of the time at Travencore is spent lying stretched out in sleep with insufficient waking hours to appreciate the novel comfort of these quarters.

Tomorrow there will be a delay in settling into our daytime sleep. King George VI has died suddenly and we are to attend a memorial service at St James' Church. We are instructed to collect a black armband from Matron's office before marching the short distance along Macquarie Street.

I also learned this morning Barbara's night duty has been postponed following a painful accident, and I feel for her. Unwell, with associated vomiting, she fainted returning from the bathroom at the Young Street Annexe. As she fell, face down, her two front teeth were knocked out by contact with the edge of a step. When found, the nerve endings were hanging down in the empty space where her teeth should have been. She phoned Matron later in the day explaining the accident and her inability to go on night duty that night. The response was a deep sigh then the irritable reply:

'This is very inconvenient Nurse. It will be difficult to replace you at this late stage.'

18

Routines, Comparisons and the Unthinkable

The hanging contents of the wardrobe are skimmed through several times. What to wear! I survey my image in the mirror, holding the garments up against me, one by one, critical of everything I pull out and replace. Finally I choose a full, patterned dirndl skirt with tight waistband and a close-fitting white blouse. My watch is checked too often, and the hands never seem to move at the correct pace, so I sit on the bed and wait.

Rehoused at Young Street following night duty, with four days' leave starting tomorrow, at any moment the front door bell should ring and William will be shown into the Visitors' Sitting Room. I have not laid eyes on him for 15 months. It is impossible to bring to mind a clear picture of his face: his features are a blur, only recalled when I look at his photo, framed and standing on the dressing table. He won't have heard from me for three months. Due to his rushed packing and getting away from Fraserburgh, he has forgotten to send the name and postal address of Blue Funnel's shipping agents in South Africa. A telephone conversation received this morning following connection of the ship-to-shore telephone, his soft Aberdonian accent heard again, my excited reply was short. All will soon be conveyed face to face and I give directions to Young Street. Perhaps I should have met the *Diomed* at Walsh Bay after checking the arrival time and place of berthing in the Herald, but instead I merely hung about in a state of nervous excitement knowing he would telephone.

There it is at last, the metal burr of the front entrance bell and, although the sound is expected, I jump. The creak of the front door opening and Sister Campbell's voice is calling my name up the stairs. Checking my hair in the mirror, another spray of perfume just for luck, I'm not conscious of descending to the floor below but hear the resonance of my click-clacking heels on the austerely covered stairs.

Entering the open doorway into the sitting room, immediately the smile so well remembered lights up his face.

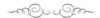

The interminable train journey I criticised the previous spring is not long enough now, with my head resting on William's shoulder and his arm around me through the night hours, until I wake with the grinding of slowing wheels when the train slides alongside Wauchope station. We alight and turn towards the exit leading into the car park.

The air is hot and motionless shimmering above the small town. The stationmaster, hoping to compensate for the treeless lack of shade surrounding the building and conscious of his station's presentation to its passengers, has placed staghorns at intervals around the outside walls. Their fronds droop sadly as though fretting for their rainforest birthplace or a cool ocean breeze, which does not reach this far from the coast. My father is waiting in his utility—half an hour to the sea and a warm welcome home.

A term of surgical nursing lectures is a grounding for the approaching period in Ward 12, a women's surgical area, situated in the Renwick Pavilion on the hospital's southern boundary. The extended light and airy space is obviously busy, and increasingly so as the day wears on, which is reflected in the working sounds. Surgical trays and trolleys being set up near the entrance; steam clouds gushing up out of opened steriliser lids; rumbling screens pulled and pushed; meals being served; and doctors and nurses voicing instructions to each other and patients. It's not long before 8.15 a.m. arrives, ushering in the tall Sister-in-charge, graced with a regal bearing and a cool, verging on cold, persona. I decide keeping my head down and getting on with the job is the best way to proceed. It proves to be too busy to do other than concentrate on the morning's work. Preparing patients listed for theatre during the afternoon, I begin at the beginning, mentally ticking off tasks as I go.

Depending on the operation site and whether internal or external, certain preparations are routine and necessary. Shavings of pure soap are stirred vigorously into an aluminium enema can containing warm water, the temperature checked, and the apparatus is held at the nurse's shoulder height. The frothy liquid obeys the force of gravity spiralling downwards through the rubber tubing; a tiny bakelite tap turned on allows the contents into the rectal tube, fulfilling its purpose.

Pubic or underarm hair and a substantial surrounding area is shaved then skin preparation is carried out with careful attention to asepsis; sterile towels are arranged around the exposed operation area; sterile forceps and cotton wool are used to swab the skin with various lotions. Ethereal soap, applied working out from the centre, with attention to the umbilicus, is washed off with sterile water, followed by the application of assorted antiseptic lotions. As I apply the final touch, wrapping a sterile drawsheet around the patient's abdomen and pinning it securely with sterile pins, I am reminded of the story told by theatre staff after the homeless eccentric, Bea Miles was wheeled into theatre, already anaesthetised, then placed on the operating table. The safety pins undone and the sterile sheet unwrapped, a note fell out and lay on Bea's bacteria-free abdomen. It read 'Please leave something behind'.

I do not envisage these lengthy preparations being simplified or abandoned. They are an essential series of steps to be carried out for the patient's welfare.

The anaesthetist's prescribed premedication is derived from drugs prepared in tablet form or sometimes supplied in ampoules. A tablet is placed on a pre-boiled spoon; sterile water is drawn into the syringe, expelled onto the tablet, and drawn up and expelled until the tablet is properly dissolved, then checked by Sister. Carefully stored warnings locked into my brain react and remind me:

Needles need frequent sharpening

Check that the patient is the correct recipient

Never use a blunt needle

Expel air from the syringe, which, according to Modern Practical Nursing Procedures, may cause an embolus (clot) if injected into a blood vessel, with sudden death following (though the book thankfully adds that this is a rare occurrence), then the hypodermic injection can be administered.

Syringe and needle must be rinsed, boiled and stored ready for re-use, in a purpose-designed, covered tray, filled with methylated spirits.

The patient en route from theatre to ward must be carefully observed following the anaesthetist's final check in the corridor outside theatre, where the patients recover. The journey back to the safety of his or her bed can be fraught with unexpected occurrences, or in my case an absolute expectation of dramatic incidents, before this duty becomes routine.

Walk at the head of the trolley. Don't rush and don't allow the theatre orderly to rush. Keep a close eye on the patient's colour for a change to blue, sometimes hard to discern when passing through dark passageways, especially after dark in a hospital with dingy corners and dimly lit thoroughfares. If there is an insufficient airway, bring the patient's jaw forward by placing the fingers below the ear and behind the angle of the jaw. Often a Guedel airway is in place, held in position by a rubber flange that fits over the lips, connected to a passageway for air that rests on the tongue.

I carry the 'anaesthetic' tray, which consists of a kidney dish containing instruments that may have to be used; a mouth gag, placed to keep the mouth open, sponge-holding forceps, swabs and tongue forceps of barbaric appearance, which I hope I will never have to apply in retrieving a tongue fallen back into the pharynx, blocking the airway. The metal spike at the point of the forceps, shaped like a canine eye-tooth, is clamped into the tongue's tip and drawn forward—though it must be remembered that less damage will be inflicted on the tongue if the forceps are inserted horizontally and not vertically through the tip.

If it comes to the crunch, send the theatre attendant for help. It is all explained in our *Tutor School Bible* and written by those stalwart Sisters, Doherty, Sirl and Ring.

Upon arrival of the trolley in the ward, I screen the prepared operation bed, remove the three weighty, barrel-shaped, ceramic hot-water bottles, assist with lifting the patient into a warmed bed and add the extra comfort of a hot blanket. The Guedel airway will be removed and the patient placed in a semi-prone position when fully conscious.

Observation, the No. 11 Indispensable Quality Required in the Nurse, is now given priority. It is a necessary skill acquired in watching for objective and subjective signs, adding a valuable aid to the doctor's assessment of his patient. At his discretion the new antibiotic, penicillin, a remarkable therapeutic success, may be ordered if infection is likely.

The anaesthetists' order for post-operative pain, pethidine or morphine sulphate, is administered. For the extreme pain of terminal cases heroin is known to be prescribed.

The first morning in Ward 12 worked through, this is the afternoon in the week when the five of us attend a compulsory six-week course in invalid cookery. Our return to Young Street and relaxation—dragging off the oppressive uniform, soiled apron and hot black stockings, kicking off shoes, removing the cap and shaking out the hair, followed by a soothing shower, have to be postponed. We are chauffeured to and from East Sydney Technical College in a hospital car, where pupils and teacher endure several hours of instruction. We prepare dishes under her supervision: a cuisine of tripe, blancmange, colourless puddings, eggnog and white sauce. With the exception of beef tea, every dish presented is an insipid colour. If one person finds some small item or word humorous it triggers an episode of uncontrollable giggling, expected of teenagers, not 21-year-old women. Laughter acts like a relief valve after a morning's tiring and sometimes emotional ward work, but it is tough on the teacher. As we file out on the last day, she assures us we are the most inattentive and silly group she has come across, but we feel no shame.

During her training at St Thomas's before their adventurous voyage south, Miss Osburn learnt to prepare a cuisine of 'sick cooking'. The easy to swallow porridge, egg flips and puddings must contain wonderful properties — more than 80 years later, in the 1950s, we have prepared an identical menu for the invalid.

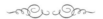

The Prince Edward in Castlereagh Street is an impressive cinema built in the grand picture palace style. The usherettes, smartly decked out in uniform, are showing patrons to numbered seats allotted at the box office. To the right of the stage the steadfast Noreen Hennessy, with feet flying right then left on the Wurlitzer organ's pedals, creates a tremendous sound that soars up into the auditorium's rafters. At the close of the five o'clock session, over one of Cahill's soda fountain specialities, William reveals he has obtained a position as a seagoing engineer, and when I realise the significance of this, my spirits take a dive. I envisage more long separations, weeks at a time, until he quickly continues.

'I've been offered the Second Engineer's position on board the Wallarah, one of the sixty milers.' Seeing the puzzled look on my face, he explains. 'Small colliers that carry coal from Newcastle to Sydney, a distance of 64 nautical miles, hence the name. It means I will be home every other night and it will suit us both. They are distinctive on the harbour with their elongated funnels and nothing much to spare above the load line when returning filled with coal.'

I begin to smile showing how pleased I am for him, knowing his love for the sea, and that this will be enough to keep that love satisfied.

'They are part of a great tradition dating back to the early 1800s, when sailing ships carried the coal. I'm sure to be able to point one out to you on our next ferry ride,' he concludes.

I am happy that things are working out for him, just as he has been lucky to find decent digs at Neutral Bay. After all, he has given up his home and career to come back to me, thousands of sea miles working under difficult conditions.

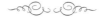

Yesterday's happenings are still in my mind as I approach the Nurses' Dining Room before the start of the 2 p.m. shift. I am surprised no-one is seated at the tables. The room is empty except for a solitary maid standing desolately at the doorway.

'Where is everyone?' I ask, eyeing the area usually overflowing with chattering nurses at this time.

'Didn't you hear?' the maid shows surprise. 'The nurses are boycotting the dining room today and won't be coming in for meals.'

'I haven't heard anything about it.'

'They are on strike because of the food. Not good enough they say.'

Pulling out a chair at the nearest table I sit down. Then I vaguely remember hearing a rumour a few weeks earlier that this might happen, but who would have organised it and how would I have known about it? It isn't something anyone would dare to add to the glass-enclosed noticeboard. It must have been circulated by word of mouth during my day off.

Self-preservation clicks in and now that I am seated I may as well eat. It will be a long afternoon and evening without food, and even if I had more than the few pence rolling around in my money purse, there isn't enough time to slip out and downtown to buy the cheapest meal I know—a few slices of raisin toast. A few minutes pass before I lift my knife and fork to begin eating the usual unappetising meal the maid has set in front of me. Slight feelings of guilt felt one moment are alternating with thoughts of self-interest as I appease my hunger.

Suddenly there is a loud clatter of descending footsteps on the cedar staircase. Matron has heard the news. Her white figure pauses a few steps from the bottom, enabling her to survey the deserted dining room. She cannot avoid noting my solitary presence but gives no sign of recognition. Fury has blurred her vision I decide, fork poised in front of my mouth, as Matron's face grows livid, a rosy spot flaring on each cheek. She turns abruptly and retraces her steps. Her veil bristles as she moves up the stairs with an agility that is astonishing, considering Matron must be at least sixty.

By the following afternoon the air has cleared, although Matron's fierce figure is not sighted. She has made it clear through a curt notice placed on the noticeboard that she does not approve of strike action or any revolt against authority or anybody associated with the same, and rebellion is an undesirable quality in any nurse. The nurses made an attempt to air their disapproval of the unsuitable food provided. There is no organising body to assist in their complaint and their effort produces scant improvement.

It is rumoured that Matron Pidgeon is severely taken aback at the nurses' decision to take some action, albeit a minor one. She trained in an even stricter era, and served in the army during a war where disobedience was unthinkable. Her expectations of her nurses are similar: humbly follow routine; question nothing; accept what is given without question; obey seniors without resentment; and above all, first and last, remember that nursing is the giving of self. Nurses understand this is the way it is, but the body requires more. Edible sustenance is essential in coping with hard work and long hours.

19

Your Place or Mine

'So, the woman I love is a scab.'

After hearing my account of the nurses' boycott of the dining room and laughing heartily, William's mirth intensifies the blue of his eyes as I sip my coffee and study his face over the rim of the cup.

'Scab. What a horrible description,' I answer indignantly. 'It has all kinds of connotations, particularly to a nurse. And what does it really mean?'

William explains that a scab is one who refuses to strike or tries to break a strike by continuing to work. He keeps on smiling, adding reassuringly, 'The word has no connection with you. A stupid description I could not in all seriousness apply to you,' and he squeezes my hand.

'Anyhow,' I reply, 'I was not on duty at the time and I was exceedingly hungry.'

I am pleased that he doesn't point out that although not on duty I had defied the veto, and quickly changing the subject he asks, 'What would you like to do this evening?'

No matter how we choose to fill in the rest of the afternoon and evening, and I with my late pass, it will be agreeable for both of us, as long as it is spent together. Where we spend the evening's end and the saying of goodnight affords us small choice. There is no shelter available where we can be alone together. His home is a rented room in someone else's house, shared with a friendly but curious family. My residence is akin to a nunnery. The evening invariably ends with us seated on our favoured park bench, beneath a Morton Bay fig behind the Conservatorium of Music.

'Let's get married soon. And I mean soon,' I whisper as we sit quietly, arms around each other, holding onto the warmth of the other's body, preventing that comfort from escaping on the rapidly cooling night air.

'There is nothing I look forward to more than that.' William places a kiss on my forehead. 'And it will happen. But you would have to resign and waste three years of training. Just another 12 months to go and we will marry as we planned. In the end you won't regret it and may even be pleased that you've achieved what you set out to do.'

I know he is right—always positive with his usual touch of humour, exactly what I rely on to guide me through the final 12 months. Traffic sounds are lessening. The rustle of nesting birds overhead and their occasional shrill cry diminish. The stars are blacked out behind low-level cloud moving in over the city.

Standing, we turn towards the line of streetlights casting a soft glow along Macquarie Street, then cross for the short walk to the Young Street Annexe.

An unexpected privilege improves our social life when Sister Campbell calls me by name as I return to my room after morning tea. Half-way up the staircase I hesitate, then step back down the stairs to meet the Home Sister. She takes hold of my hand and presses a key into my palm.

'Keep this,' she whispers. 'It is a key to the front door. Use it when you need to come in late,' and placing a finger to her lips turns her head to look behind, but there is no-one else in the corridor. The widespread wings of her white veil, so well starched, make a faint scraping sound as they move across her uniformed shoulders.

'Use it with care,' she continues. I am positive this means don't allow Sister Galway, the head Home Sister, to catch me turning the key in the lock.

'Your young man is such a pleasant person,' and it flashes through my mind that dear, sweet, Sister Campbell is biased because William is a Scot.

Wearing slacks is not allowed when off duty, either within the hospital precincts or when dressed to leave the nurses' home. The comfort of wearing trousers is customary for me, admiring and copying my mother who is slim and straight backed in her daffodil coloured one-piece linen pants suit. It is a simple matter to wear slacks when going out for those nurses whose homes are in the city, and I do so by slipping out through the front door dressed in my pants suit while Sister Galway is not in sight. Rarely up late, Sister Galway will be sleeping soundly in her hairnet and bed socks on the top floor when I return, stealing in after midnight with the use of my key.

'Unsuitably attired,' says the doorman, as I stand feeling embarrassed, dressed in my tartan pants suit beside William at the entrance to the Rex Hotel lounge in King's Cross, and I feel the flush spreading over my cheeks. We find a more welcoming atmosphere in an unlicensed downstairs coffee shop further along the street where alcohol can be ordered if the patron doesn't mind drinking out of a coffee cup.

20

Broken Bones and Dented Dignity

Standing at the door and viewing the length of Ward 9, the male fracture ward, I see that a few beds of one type cluster together like becalmed sailing ships. The perpendicular struts of the frames form masts; the horizontal beams are spars; a rigging of ropes, pulleys and weights are used in traction; leather and metal constitute a Thomas's splint; the sails made of sheeting are furled and secured over bed cradle frames; and wooden blocks under the front bed end anchor the vessel to keep the cargo of broken hips from shifting.

The ward is mainly filled with heavy patients, which makes a busy workload, so that at the end of my first week I am inclined to wish the 20 beds would sail out through the door, carrying their shipment of fractured femurs, broken humerus bones, cracked spines, and the split clavicle, scapula, radius, ulna, tibia and fibular.

Several wardsmen stationed in the ward assist with lifting patients, erecting or disassembling bed frames, and other heavy duties, as well as the care of patients held in the four-bed side

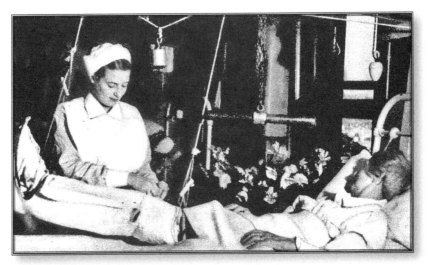

Attending a patient in a female fracture ward. (Pix *magazine, courtesy of Mitchell Library, State Library of NSW, 1940)*

room, a darkened room reserved for severe cases suffering a fractured skull. When I first enter this confined space my impressions are of an eerie and haunting scene. Suddenly I am overcome by a feeling of claustrophobia, but out of necessity it is just as quickly banished.

Strangely inhuman sounds circle in the gloom over beds enclosed in cot sides and a canvas restriction sheet that is stretched and fastened across the top to prevent these poor confused patients from climbing out and inflicting further trauma on themselves. Cot sides rattle; guttural groans emerge; and occasionally shouts or curses are heard. One patient lies in a phase of snoring on his back, and occasionally one may crawl around like a trapped animal in his cage. The initial stage of observation is possibly followed by surgical treatment, the neurosurgeon performing a craniotomy to relieve pressure on the brain. The wardsman's nursing assistance in changing a soiled bed or in preparing a patient for theatre is a valued aid.

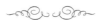

Shifts allotted to me during this period in Ward 9 do not coincide with any arrival of a patient transferred from Casualty into the 'shock bed'. There is no anguished wailing of a siren down the full length of the driveway from the hospital gates to the door of Casualty and no phone call from that department's Charge Sister alerting the ward to the impending arrival of a seriously traumatised patient. Nor will I witness the arrival of a trolley escorted by Casualty medical and nursing staff and an extra influx of doctors thrusting through the ward doors. I have no wish to experience assisting in the crush of staff around a bedside already attended by adequate personnel. Instead I am happy not to have any interruption to my ward routine with everything flowing satisfactorily as it is at this moment. There are often feelings of frustration in any ward, when procedures cannot be followed exactly as taught and demonstrated, due to staff shortages.

The patients' evening meal has been served by Sister from the hot trolley sent up from the kitchen. She sets an example of serving the food neatly onto plates; gravy spills are wiped from crockery edges with a clean tea towel. Drinks will be served with cups and glasses filled no further than an inch from the top. This is so well drilled into me I know I will spend the rest of my life following this pattern.

Face, hands and back of bed patients are sponged, the ward tidied and bedclothes straightened by my two junior nurses. Sister has finished her day at 6 p.m., and I switch on the ward lights as daylight fades. The hands on the ward clock indicate seven o'clock, and I pull back the ward doors and secure them. A sea of visitors' faces greets me, but then look expectantly beyond me, searching for a glimpse of a relative or friend before filing into the ward.

My junior nurses are sent to supper in the Nightingale Wing, and I set about the preparation for changing dressings after visiting hour. Most patients are cheerful, younger survivors of misadventure caused by motor bike or car accidents, work injuries, football clashes and other risk-taking pastimes in which males like to involve themselves.

The inevitable interruptions occur: requests for urinals, changing a patient's position or adjusting an aching limb among the fractured femurs.

The evening nursing supervisor is due to arrive, which necessitates my accompanying her on a round of the patients and answering questions about their condition.

Preoccupied with setting up trays and avoiding the clouds of searing steam rising out of the steriliser, set to scald my face, my thoughts are already on my next task. This area, situated to the left of the entrance, is open to the ward, so I can watch over the patients at the same time.

I am unaware of Sister's presence until I hear her voice and the chilly tone in the words spoken.

'Nurse, are you aware that your juniors are out in the day room drinking beer with the wardsmen?'

Startled, my body shaking, I spin around, dropping the kidney dish into the boiling water sending droplets of heat spraying up and stinging my bare arms. Out of the corner of my eye I see the two shame-faced nurses return to the ward where they begin the nightly round of removing and folding the bed quilts.

There is a long moment of silence while I take in the seriousness of Sister's words and her obvious vexation as she waits with a cross expression clouding her face and one corner of her mouth twitching.

'No, I didn't know,' I pull myself together, gather up a dressing towel and wipe my smarting arms.

'I sent them to supper and naturally thought they had left the ward.'

'I will have to report this to Matron. You are in charge and she will question how this came about and why you were not aware

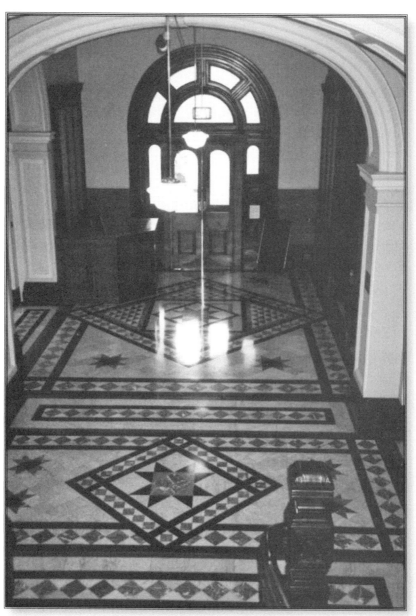
Entrance foyer of the administration building, Sydney Hospital, 2008. (Author photograph)

of it. After all, the day room is quite close by.'

What is the point of trying to explain—the involvement in my work with one nurse less than usual or that it is improper to leave the ward unattended. My explanations and how I will present them are already filling my head in readiness for the call to Matron's office.

Sister's veil disappears out into the corridor and my fury and embarrassment surface. I feel betrayed by the silly juniors, taking advantage with their unprofessional behaviour. Even worse, the patients will be made aware of their lack of sobriety when alcoholic fumes are breathed in their faces. I rein in my anger, while they do their utmost to stay out of my way.

The call to Matron's office hasn't eventuated. Instead, a summons to a higher authority is received.

The Medical Superintendent's office is located in the centre administration building, entered from Macquarie Street by imposing stone stairs or as I have, by coming from the interior hospital buildings, across the adjoining arched sandstone bridges. No-one else is in the foyer, except the attendant standing behind a desk near the front entrance. Following his directions I cross the black and white tiled floor, passing by the solid marble honour rolls framed in the ubiquitous mahogany and topped with a pediment. An elegant carved staircase leads up to a landing and stained glass memorial windows. I rarely see this area, which, built to impress, has the same ambience as a church interior, suggesting the voice must not be raised above a whisper.

The door, with the occupant's title painted in gold letters, is partially open and I knock gently at exactly 2 p.m., the time of my appointment. A voice answers giving permission to enter. Dr Norman Rose is known to me and all trainees, due to our brief encounters on his midnight rounds with the Night Sister when he questions our knowledge on patients and equipment, with the occasional trick question on world affairs thrown in. His head is raised from the paperwork spread across his desk and I am told to take a seat. To rest the weakness in my knees and balance uneasily on the edge of the chair is a relief. He has a reputation that describes him as a reasonable man, without the god-like persona of some of the older Honorary Medical Officers visiting the wards. It is also known he had served in the war for five years, taking leave a year after he commenced as Superintendent, and returning to the position in 1945. Dr Rose straightens and leans back in his cumbersome office chair. I detect a twinkle in his eye, so I relax a little.

'Well, Nurse MacSkimming, tell me your side of the episode when you were in charge of Ward 9 two evenings ago and your nurses were found to be consuming alcohol.'

I calmly relate my version, hoping that Matron has passed on a reasonable recommendation of my past training so far, if anything of that nature has been requested.

Dr Rose's verdict is given like a judge, but not a severe one, saying he finds my explanation reasonable, summing up with: 'Ward 9 is a busy ward and often requires many things to be dealt with at one time.' He pauses and puts my face under close scrutiny. 'You have a very satisfactory record and the ward is waiting. I'm sure there will be duties unattended in your absence and needing your care.'

Swivelling his chair to one side he prepares to stand indicating that the interview is over. I am thankful on quitting the office, with its old-fashioned Victorian fustiness, and ignore the two culprits waiting and looking sheepish in the corridor. I hope Dr Rose will show some severity towards them, with none of the understanding he gave me. This is not the time for acknowledgment, and I hurry back across the entrance foyer.

Relating this experience to William, always an interested listener, I explain that I'm unsure why the Medical Superintendent has questioned me and why it was not under Matron's jurisdiction as Head of Nursing. Nursing and Medical were separately managed. Shrugging my shoulders I answer the question myself. Perhaps it goes beyond Matron, with the Medical Superintendent responsible for overall hospital infringements of any nature if deemed serious enough.

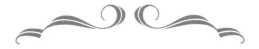

Another Thorn in the Side

Irritates and tests ... *Miss Osburn's habitually serene expression is replaced by one of annoyed vexation.*

Standing before Lucy's desk, Sister Eliza Blundell's face is more than a match for that of her superior. Eyes glaring, Eliza is prepared to brazen it out and, observing this, Lucy is reminded to include a description of Eliza's personality changes in her next letter to Miss Nightingale—how her mood swings can suddenly alter like the chameleon's ability to abruptly adapt another disguise. She intends to emphasise just how trying this is.

Further back in time, which now seems to be decades ago instead of two years, first impressions of Eliza were of a good, practical nurse with a lively intelligence. An Anglican widow, she has developed the same embarrassing behaviour with the opposite sex as Annie and Bessie, although Miss Osburn is of the opinion intelligence is not a drawcard for most men. Eliza has copied her colleagues in indulging in flirtatious relationships with men. Indeed, Bessie Chant had caused much gossip with the outcome of her affair with a man, falling pregnant and forced to resign. Florence Nightingale and Lucy deeply disapproved of this behaviour and seemed to expect the Nightingale nurses' to follow a career in nursing, not marrying.

Which brings Lucy to another point she must raise in her letter. That is the false belief, voiced by Miss Wardroper, that if the nurses chosen for Sydney were over 30, they would be too old to be migrating in the hope of finding a husband.

'It has come to my attention that two men are vying for your affections. One, I believe, is a patient, and the other is a member of staff.' Here Miss Osburn hesitates, then concludes on a higher note in

disbelief, 'A wardsman?'

She presses on, 'I also have been told that you allow them to visit your bedroom. Do you think this behaviour is suited to a Nightingale nurse?'

At least Annie Miller's experimental love affair, while privately entertaining a male in her room, was spent with a Resident Medical Officer, a person of higher status.

Eliza's eyes are concealed behind narrow slits in her grim face. Lucy has seen this expression build on other occasions, and hopes that this will not develop into one of her violent temper tantrums, often accompanied by the use of foul language and quite shocking.

Drawing in a deep breath and making an obvious effort to control her reactions, Eliza's eyes reappear and colour returns to her cheeks. 'Yes, I am hostess to friends who occasionally join me in my room and we chat, over the sharing of a pot of tea. I can see no harm in that, Miss Osburn.'

The ever-watchful Haldane Turiff has reported that the beverage is of a stronger nature.

'If this entertaining involves alcohol then you must desist, Eliza. Your role requires dignity at all times, setting an example for the trainee nurses. I place great importance on the Sisters and the Nurses being models of sobriety.'

Following the interview Miss Osburn opens a desk drawer and takes out next week's roster. The scratching pen moves Sister Blundell to a female ward, where there is no likelihood of encounters with wardsmen or male patients.

She throws the sheets of paper back into the drawer with vigour and slams it shut.

Lucy's patience, like a spiderweb stretched to the limit and fragile, has held fast in the face of a rising storm.

21

Milestones Celebrated

The fourth-year cap is a more feminine version of the third-year model. Lace, the pattern chosen by the wearer, is sewn around the edge of the three scallops forming the band; another step in the four years and a sign that there is light at the end of the tunnel. A date is being set for the Hospital Nursing Staff Celebratory Ball. The importance of what to wear is an ongoing discussion, along with the topic of who to ask as a partner. My choice is a foregone conclusion.

'We are so looking forward to the ball. The date has been set and the venue decided—the Great Hall of Sydney University.' Taking hold of William's arm we set off up Young Street towards the city centre.

'Sounds very impressive.'

'Be sure to have that night arranged to spend ashore.'

'Of course,' William replies with a grin. 'I will jump overboard and swim to land if necessary.'

On arrival at the Nurses' Annexe, William always stands in Bridge Street looking up at the bedroom window and whistling sharply. Seeing my face behind the glass pane and my hand waving in answer, he lifts his hat and smiles. On the night of the ball, being such a special occasion, he rings the doorbell and waits in the stark Visitors' Sitting Room. Sister Campbell is quick to compliment him on his appearance and I must agree: he is the perfect gentleman in dinner suit, red bow tie with matching handkerchief peaks showing above his coat pocket, and shoes shone to perfection, a meticulous habit of his. I burst into the room flushed with excitement and swirl around, creating the satisfying sound of rustling taffeta beneath the voile evening dress. William is waiting for me to settle before pinning an orchid corsage onto my bodice.

The taxi pulls up in the gravel driveway before the Great Hall's Gothic splendour. A shaft of light from the open doorway splits the darkness, and high stone ramparts are silhouetted against the starry sky. Sounds of laughter and the band already in full swing indicate dancing is in progress. Our table is located, greetings exchanged, introductions made. All my friends have arrived and we are soon mingling with those on the crowded dance floor.

The following day a post mortem is held on the previous evening's success and, encouraged by our laughter, Pat describes how holding her partner's hand, circling quickly under his extended arm he inadvertently placed his foot on her full length gown. A movement acted out at a speed too fast for the restricted strapless dress and built in bra, they were prevented from turning with her, revealing more than she would have wished.

Our elevated spirits heightened by the good feeling of a memorable evening are quickly banished when news speeds through the hospital. In the early morning hours after the ball an accident took place. Two recently married Sisters were killed in a horrific car smash. At that stage it is not known if their husbands have survived.

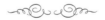

The droning of a blowfly puts the seal on the authenticity of a perfect summer day. The insect tries desperately to gain the warm air outside, perhaps to set a course for the harbour's blue serenity nearby. Unable to escape, the fly is bent on committing suicide with a succession of attempts by battering its head against the windowpane.

'How the hell did that thing get in here?' growls the ophthalmic surgeon as the scout nurse administers the death blow with a rolled-up towel. I shudder. I have seen the results of a blowfly's habits and the fulfilment of its purpose in life by depositing its young in the perfect environment. A fan whirrs noiselessly in one corner of the small operating theatre, making little impression in the stuffy air. Someone comments across the operating table how perfect the day is and how pleasant for those out there enjoying the sunshine. The one least aware of the afternoon's beauty is the waiting patient stretched out in the middle of this group in a preliminary sedated state.

I envy the scout nurse's flexibility in moving around the enclosed room, while I am confined to remaining stock still throughout the third cataract extraction on the operation list. A stool supports me where I stand opposite the Surgeon and Theatre Sister. My role is to keep as still as possible and train a hand-held light onto the operation field. It requires a steady hand and a settled stomach as the surgeon injects local anaesthetic, the upper and lower eyelids held open by a retractor.

The atmosphere in the theatre is quiet as an incision is made. It is essential that the light remain without movement and I concentrate with all the attentiveness I can muster. I must be trying too hard, with rigid fingers holding the handle in a vice-like grip and my eyes beginning to ache. The circle of light is growing fuzzy, quivering over the operation site. My knees turning to jelly as I go down, I glimpse a blurred image of the surgeon, lifting his eyes and scalpel simultaneously.

'Quick, grab her!' he bellows.

Somebody moves smartly and grasps my hand and the light

before I lay myself across the patient's torso. When I fully regain my equilibrium in an anteroom I am not expected to return to the theatre. I don't feel foolish when later I learn this is a frequent occurrence.

Sydney Eye Hospital is situated in Sir John Young Crescent, Woolloomooloo. The 1885 building was originally constructed as an alcohol-free hotel, referred to as a 'coffee palace' and named Pacific Mansions. In 1922, under the auspices of Sydney Hospital, it became the Sydney Eye Hospital. The late nineteenth-century building has the musty atmosphere occasionally associated with ageing Victorian establishments. An outpatients' department is on the ground floor, and the floors above are divided into gloomy rooms for nursing inpatients recovering from eye trauma and surgery.

On return to one of these wards at the end of surgery, Mr Burgess, who was so briefly placed under my spotlight, is carefully lifted into bed. A nurse steadies his head and a sandbag is placed beside each ear to prevent movement, which also means the rest of his body is restricted and he will be nursed in that position for three weeks. When fully conscious he is warned not to sneeze, cough or touch his bandaged eyes. I feed him, attend to his toilet and, with assistance, turn him to care for his back. A complication for these elderly patients is delirium. The night nurse reports that Mr Burgess experienced an unsettled night, woke confused in the blacked out night hours, his disorientation compounded by bandaged eyes. He pulled off his dressings, attempted to get out of bed and was difficult to settle despite heavy sedation. At the close of three long weeks the operation is pronounced successful, despite his disturbed nights. This coincides with my move into another phase of training.

'I am dreading Monday,' I confess over my shoulder before stepping off the moving escalator and waiting for William.

'Of course you do, I know you and your dislike of changing to another area.' He gives my hand a squeeze as we walk the length of the shopping arcade. 'But I know how well you will cope despite your fears. Think of something pleasant, concentrate on what we are about to do.' Thoughts and doubts about the coming week and introduction to the main hospital's operating theatres are pushed to the back of my mind.

I rarely shop in Her Majesty's Arcade, one of several running between streets in the city centre. The rows of shopfront windows are filled with fashionably attired store dummies, and the premises leased mainly to newly arrived European migrants. Their selling techniques are full of overwhelming assurances that every garment tried on, no matter how unsuitable, is perfect for that buyer and in the end, confused, I am glad to escape their persistence.

We are on the verge of making a once in a lifetime purchase as we approach the jeweller's at the far end of the top floor. This level has a dull appearance, gloomily lit, the site of workshops for tradesmen and wholesalers working behind opaque windows with few displays. There is no pressure from this salesman, only patience as together we choose a single diamond set in gold and platinum, a ring within William's price range.

'Do you want to wear it now?' the jeweller asks, before slipping the ring back into the box and closing the lid with a sharp snap.

'No, not until the dinner party when it will be made official.'

An occasion happily anticipated and another reason not to dwell on Sister Hundt's reputation for icy supervision of that unknown quantity, the isolated world of starkly tiled operating theatres.

Three close friends accompanied by partners share our celebration with dinner and dancing at Carl Thomas's on the following Saturday. It is a well-known nightclub, within walking distance at the harbour end of Macquarie Street, and housed in a row of solid nineteenth-century wool stores facing across Circular

Quay to their counterparts on the western shore in the shadow of the Harbour Bridge. The top floor conversion has been kept to a minimum. A high wide aperture, once open to enable wool bales to be swung out and down to the waiting horse-drawn carts below, is now permanently enclosed. The hardwood walls block out the nightscape; light dances on the harbour's moving surface and illuminated ferries slide in and out of the Circular Quay wharves. No regret is expressed at the lack of an outlook. Our group is more interested in drinking and dancing encircled in our partners' arms, until the clock signals the evening's close and an escape into the clear night air, away from the pall of cigarette smoke stinging our eyes.

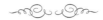

The high-pitched shrilling shatters my deep sleep. I roll over quickly and turn the alarm off. Not due on duty until this afternoon, Barbara's curled up form in the opposite bed does not stir. Quietly dressing, tying my cap in position, the final important detail is addressed: I remove my diamond ring, slide it onto a safety pin and secure it in my breast pocket. By the time the hospital car delivers the Young Street group inside the Macquarie Street gates I am fully awake. A cup of tea and a cigarette in the Nightingale Wing's basement should help to settle my stomach, but instead sends it into a frenzied rumbling.

'How can you smoke at this hour?' asks one of the few non-smokers, as I draw heavily on a cigarette. An unnecessary query, since almost everyone smokes at this time of the day. But I answer with the explanation that it soothes the nerves. The sun is rising behind the Domain as I follow the path leading towards the Travers block. The first rays outline the steam rising from vents on the roof above the Maitland Theatre. This early morning expulsion of steam hasn't caught my attention before, but does so now because that is my destination. The ancient lift gives a jerk then begins its reluctant climb. If I dared, for one must be careful of what one wishes, I might wish the antiquated lift rope would snap. Down we would plummet to the basement, negating the necessity to step out at the top floor and move towards the 'no unauthorised entry' sign and into the pristine white area I once glimpsed on my way to Sick Bay. The wish unfulfilled, I look for someone who will give me the first of many instructions during the next three months, plus a few warnings thrown in.

That evening, while the *Wallarah* unloads her cargo at Ball's Head, William calls from the public phone box outside the gate. During our conversation I hear the gantry crane clanging and shunting in the background as it scoops the coal out of the ship's hold and deposits it onto the loading platform.

'How did the day unfold? Was it as bad as you expected?'

'Well, no. But it was a return to the routine of my probationary year. I have washed down every tiled wall in every outside area adjacent to the theatre, high and low, and back and forth. I don't know who cleans inside the theatre but I've a feeling I know who that will be.'

William suggests dinner when next we meet and names the Normandie, one of the better restaurants in town, situated downstairs in Elizabeth Street where crumbed sole is served cooked to perfection. It will be a celebration of my survival of this first week.

'I would have given this up long ago only for you.'

I pause, adding light-heartedly, 'You have been my saviour.'

'Strong words, lass,' he is chuckling at the other end. 'That's some onus you have placed on me.'

I can picture him returning to the ship, negotiating with ease the long drop down the metal ladder attached to the sandstone wall and reaching the wharf below. Sometimes I spend the evening with him when he is required to stay on board. The *Wallarah* is a fine collier, almost new, and William's cabin is neat and comfortable, just as his cabin had been aboard *Hector*. The choice between 'his place or hers' has become his because it offers somewhere that I can join him.

22

The Other Planet

As with placement on night duty, trainees are allocated to theatre training in the order of their arrival on the first day almost four years previously. The presence of one or other of my friends close at hand or passing by in the corridors of the three main theatres makes this period much more bearable. Everyone experiences the first morning tea together, and later we can compare notes.

Each one has a different anecdote to relate, although the tense routine never varies. Sister Hundt pouring tea; the passing of cups around a circle of rigidly seated nursing staff while her dark eyes follow then rest on the newcomer, sizing her up. This penetrating look is like an order that we dare not disobey, so we accept the poured tea and drink it down, although another beverage may be preferable—or even none at all. The theatre areas in three different buildings run to perfection under her strict supervision. Nothing escapes her keen observation. She has the thin agile body of a long distance runner, ever on the move except when scrubbed and gowned working as instrument Sister beside one of the top surgeons, never missing any infringement around her and at the same time anticipating the surgeon's needs.

The first time I change into theatre garb I am careful to transfer my precious ring and pin it inside my bra. I step into the leg overalls made of thick cotton drill, pull them over my duty shoes and up over my stockings. Pinning them to my pants isn't successful. The whole invention falls down and lies over my feet. Pinning them to my suspenders and supporting suspender belt seems to work. I leave my petticoat on under the gown revealing a touch of lace at the hem. A delicate reminder of my femininity for who could guess my gender as the final touch to the disguise is added: an all-covering cap over my hair and a surgical mask to complete the outfit.

Entering a theatre for the first time with an operation in progress is like leaving the world as I know it and arriving on a strange cold planet where the language is different, with references to unknown instruments and conditions. Latin is not unfamiliar to me as it is prominent in words relating to medical terms and pharmacology and will soon be learned here.

It is the shock of the new. A tiled, sterile chamber by day, an area hosed out by night, an arena where the surgeon practises his skills and is God in his world.

The textbook demands rather than suggests that the nurse must be at all times at her post, alert and observant. Quietness is essential, at most the only one speaking is the surgeon.

In my role as dirty or scout nurse I am the one allowed to move in and out of the theatre, fetching and carrying or relaying messages while all other personnel are scrubbed, gowned and gloved, and remain on the inside until the operation concludes.

The routine quickly falls into place, and while I find it impossible not to be on the alert, I am amused that Betty and Elaine find time during their theatre experience to brush up their social arrangements. Out of the bustling mainstream traffic they find a corner or a corridor in order to exchange conversation with some member of the resident medical staff. They seem so relaxed and look delighted during this important organisation of their off-duty hours.

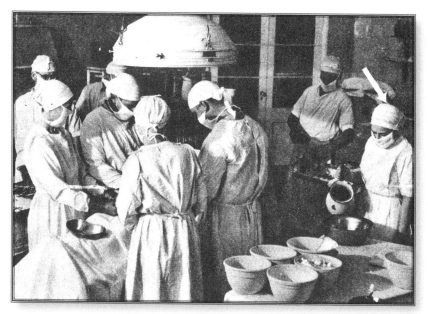

*Maitland operating theatre, Sydney Hospital, circa 1940. (*Pix *magazine, courtesy of Mitchell Library, State Library of New South Wales)*

At the completion of the day's operation list, when the theatre and surrounding areas have emptied, working a late shift and often alone, there are set tasks for the evening hours. The anterooms and theatre doors are open. The on-duty Theatre Sister is working in another theatre, and the lack of action and voices make it agreeably peaceful.

I spare a few moments to gaze out of a window facing the city's vast expanse of flickering lights. The Harbour Bridge is highlighted against the deepening navy moving in on the western sky. The lights of several craft are distinct in the vicinity. Port and masthead lights are clearly seen on a vessel before she disappears beneath the bridge heading west. I check my watch. There is a possibility of her being the *Wallarah*, due back from Catherine Hill Bay about this time, and I heave a sigh before turning back to sponge duty, an unpleasant task. Gowned and gloved I tackle the row of buckets brim-full of thickly bloodied water and soaking abdominal sponges. The pads consist of six to eight thicknesses of gauze hand-stitched together. Bending over the stainless steel sink, the size and shape reminds me of the pig trough on my uncle's farm. The sponges are washed, rinsed and squeezed out and washed again until the detritus has been removed. After an overnight soaking in a solution of Eusol they are dried and autoclaved so they will be ready to be reused.

The autoclave hisses gently in the background and I regard it with some awe the first few times I deal with it. Calico-lined metal drums contain dressings and associated accessories, placed into the barrel-like body, the large wheel is swung to secure the door and the steam pressure is raised to 10 pounds (4.5 kilograms) pressure for five minutes then 20 pounds (9.0 kilograms) for 20 minutes. When the timing is complete and the steam shut off, the drums are lifted out with forceps and the portholes quickly closed. The sterilised materials are ready for distribution throughout the wards.

The role of the trainee nurse in theatre is a subordinate one. The day is filled with cleaning, fetching, rolling bandages, making swabs from yards of cotton wool, stitching pads and being a general dogsbody. If one follows orders carefully, things usually run smoothly. Occasionally I can hover in the background and observe or look away; I choose the latter for the most part during the performance of a first-time operation in the Worral Theatre.

The theatre, cleaned and prepared meticulously under Sister Hundt's supervision, is ready well ahead of time, awaiting a prominent visiting British surgeon who is about to perform radical surgery, a hind-quarter amputation on an unfortunate young woman diagnosed with sarcoma of the right hip.

On arrival the surgeon exudes an air of extreme confidence and importance, escorted by prominent hospital surgeons surrounding him. Ever on the alert, twitching nervously in anticipation of the dramatic occasion about to unfold, Sister Hundt is in position beside the operating table and flanked by two Theatre Sisters on standby if needed. The instrument man hovers near the exit, his eyes rechecking the expanse of instruments gleaming under the circle of overhead lighting. The open-tiered gallery at the rear is filled with the many interested observers of major surgery performed by a revered surgeon.

The atmosphere is hushed as the anaesthetised patient is positioned to the surgeon's satisfaction and white figures cluster around the table. My part in this is so insignificant. I stand backed up to the western wall with little chance of seeing what is happening and, with nowhere else to look but straight ahead, I study the two circular stained glass windows set in the curved eastern wall. A touch of beauty in architect John Kirkpatrick's design; perhaps a desire to give relief and lift thoughts to a higher plane above the raw purpose of this place or maybe to insert a spiritual feel where the godly role of a saviour is entrusted to a mortal.

My drifting thoughts are jolted back into the real world when an opening appearing between two white-clad figures enables me to glimpse the surgeon's gloved hand swabbing the exposed skin area framed in sterilised sheets. There is a respectful silence as he leaves his mark on the pale skin. I am mesmerised and whereas I was unable to watch earlier, now I cannot look away. The scalpel, sharper than a razor, leaves a red trail oozing out of the incision, and the milk-white bubbles of underlying fat are exposed as the blade curves from pubic bone across the upper buttock to the base of the spine. This is accompanied by the repeated click of the assistant surgeon's artery forceps clamping blood vessels. The hushed mood in the room is occasionally broken by the surgeon's explanations of his techniques, a signal that prompts the gallery audience to push heads forward for a better view.

The primitive sound, equivalent to those of the butcher's shop, turns the stomach as the amputation saw severs the bone. The midway mark through the long process is a dull thud indicating the full-length leg and half buttock have been lifted and placed in a waiting

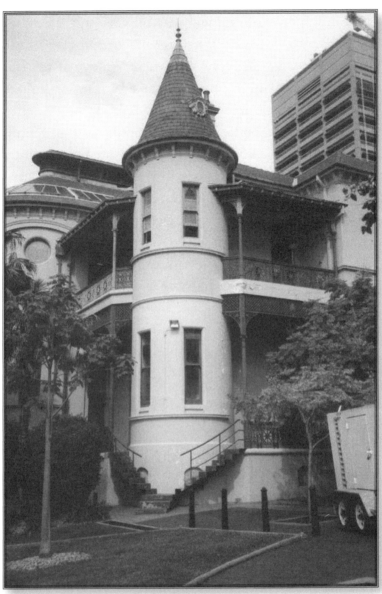

A section of John Kirkpatrick's fairytale design. Top left shows a portion of the Worral Theatre and a circular stained glass window, 2008. (Author photograph)

receptacle for delivery to Pathology, a sizable specimen transported on a covered trolley. This is my cue to creep out, not waiting to see the extent of prolonged repairs to the operation site, a skin flap applied and sutured, and the final dressing.

Seeing the young patient wheeled away to recover in the ward, I hope this procedure will save her life.

Life's alternative seems to occur mainly in the night hours. When death claims a patient, I care for the shell that remains, assisted by the relieving Night Nurse.

Death is hidden behind a closely enfolding bedscreen, glowing like a tent illuminated from within by the pale light of a torch. Death is a wax-like figure laid out and carefully attended, encased in a white shroud and labelled. The wardsman waits in the shadows beside his special trolley.

All performed quietly and quickly so that the remaining patients are unaware until, waking at daybreak, they see the bed is empty.

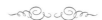

At times in theatre the laugh is at the patient's expense, happily unaware while anaesthetised. The pace is relaxed on an afternoon in the Want Theatre. Sister Hundt is darting about in the Maitland Theatre in another building, and although I admire her efficiency and am becoming accustomed to her short, sharp manner, it is better to be in the Want with a short operation list of minor cases, a pleasant gynaecologist to perform them with Sister assisting and I complying with her instructions. The surgeon is carrying out a currettage on a young girl following a miscarriage.

'This is an unusual case. A first for the textbooks,' the surgeon remarks raising his head from between the leg stirrups.

If his expression could be seen behind the surgical mask it might have shown a straight face. 'This young lady has never had sexual

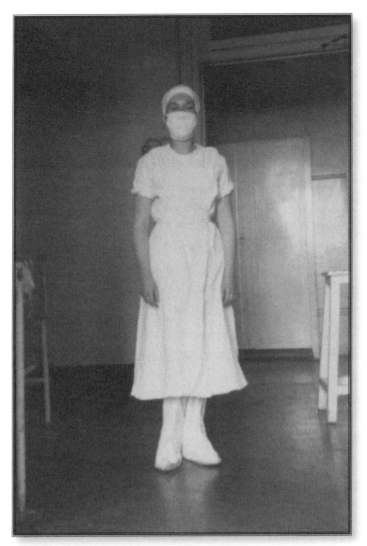

Close of long shift, Worral Theatre, October 1953. (Author photograph)

intercourse and was unlucky enough to become pregnant while sitting in her brother's bath water.'

Then the laugh was on me during a similar procedure and I, reading through the medical notes, foolishly voiced my thoughts out loud.

'The patient is not married!' I exclaim and immediately realise it was better not said. Pausing, the gynaecologist stares across the room in my direction and above her mask Sister's eyes are raised to the ceiling.

'The most unexpected things can happen in the best-regulated families. Where have you been for the past few years?'

Her rebuke is justified, but it is useless for me to try to explain that it was not my ignorance of the facts of life that caused the blunder but compassion, for there must be in every girl's mind an awareness that pregnancy outside marriage is a stigma that often results in rejection.

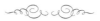

'The results are out.'

I recognise Betty's raised voice at the other end of the theatre lobby. 'We've all passed, that's the good news.' And approaching she gives a mysterious smile. 'Some better than others,' she adds.

'Don't tell me,' I quickly reply. 'I want to see for myself.'

I feel confident as I calmly scrutinise the list posted on the nurses' noticeboard shortly before 2 p.m. enabling those going on or coming off duty to see it. The results of the May Hospital Finals, which was a practice-run for the State ATNA (Australian Trained Nurses' Association) exams in October, are set out. Esme Austin's name is first on the list and she will receive the Rose Creal prize. My name is next: I was beaten by one mark.

When I complain to William about my narrow defeat, he thinks nevertheless it is a great effort and he is very proud of my achievement.

'I will receive a prize for second place. I'm not sure what that will be until the graduation ceremony in November.'

I add jokingly, 'It might be a cheque to cover all the unpaid overtime and non-existent penalty rates I might have received over recent years.' Though as a fourth year nurse, I now receive almost £3 a week. 'Just think what an acceptable start to married life that would be.'

June and her fiancé Keith marry this week in a quiet ceremony. We are sworn to secrecy, which is kept, otherwise she faces dismissal even though the end of training is only several months away.

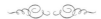

One week before returning to ward duty, I receive a phone call from Matron with the offer of a position as Acting Theatre Sister for the remainder of my training. Too surprised to say 'no', thinking it is phrased less like an offer than an order in disguise, I accept. That evening I learn Barbara has also been approached but declined, though her mother disapproves, believing it is a missed opportunity. Betty is to be the other Senior Nurse chosen to help fill the shortage of theatre staff.

This means I will be Instrument Sister for the weekly operation lists of two general surgeons, Mr Yeates and Mr Hedberg. So I begin to carry a mini-sized Theatre Instrument Manual in my pocket, referring to it, memorising it during meal breaks and other spare moments, until I feel satisfied it is glued into my brain.

The general instrument tray consists of 85 instruments, including some instruments replicated in groups, such as artery forceps. An assortment of specific instruments used for certain operations is displayed on a second tray. The sponge sister drapes the patient and is responsible for counting the pads before and after the final suturing of the wound. My responsibility, as well as anticipating and handing the surgeon the required instrument, is to count them before, then double check the count with the surgeon at the end of the operation. The instrument man whips the trays away to his work area, cleans the dirty instruments before soaking them in a 10 per cent Lysol solution and boiling them for two minutes before storing. Scalpel blades and suture needles are sharpened for reuse.

Mr Hedberg is a patient, pleasant surgeon and on first meeting is aware that I may be nervous and acknowledges my inexperienced presence by his side. Mr Yeates, with a slightly arrogant air, seems oblivious to my stand-in position. Several years later the two surgeons are fated to be leading characters in a mysterious murder. Mr Yeates will be discovered dead in his garage with signs that someone had attempted to resuscitate him. A needle had pierced the heart and perhaps the introduction of a drug used to restart the organ is an interesting disclosure. Initially Mr Hedberg was under suspicion. He later married Mrs Yeates, after a long drawn-out investigation resulted in no-one being charged.

This time of strict routine and being 'alert at my post' passes quickly and is punctuated by the ATNA exams. Luckily I am appraised at my training hospital, while some of my friends are sent to other hospitals to be examined. There is a multiple-choice paper and a viva voce, tested by a surgeon and a physician. I verbally sprint through the naming of instruments and their purpose, demonstrate the preparation of a mustard poultice, the application of bandages, set up trays and describe the stages of procedures.

Four years' apprenticeship is drawing to a close; another year of hospital statistics are tallied: we have provided a valuable service to almost 36,000 city and country dwellers.

Days off duty are happily applied to necessary tasks, planning a wedding, albeit a small affair in the country, and adding needlework and household objects to my glory box.

The final creation required in preparation for this new beginning must be quickly collected before I am due on afternoon duty—my second last. Hanging in splendid, bouffant, Swiss voile glory in the King Street dressmaker's salon, my wedding dress is complete.

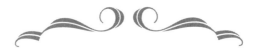

Reflections

Casting back—contemplating ... *while standing at the ward entrance in the only completed section of replacement hospital building, Miss Osburn feels a sense of pride and achievement. This is one of the few days in the past eighteen years that she feels settled, although she is very close to the end of her reign as Lady Superintendent.*

The heavily laden trunks that had arrived with her aboard ship, and a few added since, are packed and awaiting collection from her bed-sitting room. Thinking back over almost two decades there are scenes from the past still very fresh in her mind on this, her farewell inspection.

The initial demolition of the old 1811 buildings, which began almost four years before in 1881; the thud of numerous sledgehammers, crashing into unsound walls, wielded by lines of brawny labourers. Split brick and plaster tumbling in a cloud of dust. The occasional cockroach scuttling out of the debris seeking refuge in the tunnels bored through white-ant-infested wood. Cracked slate bouncing on flagstone splintering into blue-black shards. Splendid Clydesdales flex their powerful legs and stamp hair-fringed feet in time with their nodding magnificent heads as the carts stand in line waiting to take on a load before setting off southwards at a steady rate along Macquarie Street.

The Georgian-style building is slowly dying with each cartful pulled away. Filth and vermin had almost defeated the cleaning activities in these old premises but had been kept under control by sterling efforts applied under Miss Osburn's watchful eye. Lucy will not see the completed Infirmary, to be renamed Sydney Hospital, delayed in conclusion until 1894 owing to bureaucratic wrangling and the appointment of a new architect.

Standing, as always, with body erect and an expression devoid of any haughtiness, she spends some minutes observing the lilac-clad nurses bustling about their duties. She thinks about one of many obstacles following her arrival in 1868: the introduction of the delicate matter of women nursing men, which necessitated the dismissal of 12 male nurse/wardsmen, causing resentment that was finally overcome.

Recollection of difficult adversaries crowd in, one after the other, slotted into the recesses of her brain and causing disquiet, even now.

Opening the pages of every Sydney Punch *edition in trepidation, steeling herself against more slanderous articles and vicious criticism targeting herself and her reforms.*

Then came the constant opposition from Head Surgeon, Dr Roberts, who with his wife were at first valued friends. He was soon to become her enemy, opposing her on all matters. Lucy fights to keep, and wins, control over nursing, which Dr Roberts sees as his role.

'He cannot bear to see a woman in control nor in charge of any department in which he must have a complete say.'

Lucy's correspondence is like a relief valve, allowing her to get things off her chest, although proving in the long run to be unwise.

Finally, after so many years of opposition, Dr Roberts is appointed to the newly opened Royal Prince Alfred Hospital, where he is able to instigate rules Miss Osburn will not tolerate. The Matron is his subordinate, the Sisters live in rooms attached to wards and he is able to harass all levels of staff, just as he had experienced while training at Guy's Hospital in London. He informs Miss Osburn, with relish, how Sisters employed in that time were pretty young widows and very willing to wait on the Doctors.

The Royal Commission of 1873, investigating Sydney Infirmary and other public charities springs to mind. Witnesses are hostile towards her, even complaining about her personality. These complaints are rejected. The Commissioner's report is critical of all departments and systems of management in the Infirmary—except Nursing.

A faint, pleased smile touches Lucy's lips with her remembrance of the outcome and resulting dismissal of another adversary, John Blackstone, whose position as Manager is abolished.

Her inspection proceeds and she approaches other doorways in turn, leading into wards created with her ideas that patients need to be placed according to their complaints or injuries: a receiving ward of 23 beds for 'bad cases', and accident, casualty and post-operation wards.

This gives rise to thought on the doctors' interference in the teaching of her Nurses and their lectures, resentfully viewing women as incapable of studying medical subjects. They saw nurse education as a challenge to the doctors' skills and superiority, so they respond by interrupting lectures, recalling nurses to the ward where they are 'urgently needed'. One complaint is that there is too much reading to the nurses. Constant 'drilling' is the way to teach nurses.

Lucy chuckles and she pictures again the scene where she and her charges enjoy time spent at the Sisters' Sitting Room table listening to her readings on anatomy and physiology, and the interest expressed in amazing diagrams reconstructing the human body's composition and functions.

The House Visitors' Committee are at the end of their inspection as Lucy comes upon them and, beaming upon her, they pronounce a glowing report.

Extreme cleanliness and neatness are predominant; nurses' duties are attended with intelligence and thoroughness. The patients speak of their kind natures and caring attitudes.

Lucy heaves a great sigh of satisfaction. Her mind's eye creates a last scene that will remain with her for many years. Her friend Helen Lambert, arriving in the company of Lord Belmore's private secretary, not once but many times, bearing gifts of books for patients and pictures to hang, inducing a homely atmosphere.

There are no more passageways or wards to check and Lucy makes her way across the courtyard to the Nightingale Wing, passing foundations laid in readiness for the next stage of building to commence. Entering her office she closes the door for the last time and seats herself behind the imposing desk.

The drawers have been cleared of personal effects but, on the wall behind, her portrait will remain in position. All is in readiness for her successor, Sydney Infirmary graduate Rebecca McKay, to take over her role with a new title, Matron.

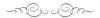

Originally signing a contract for three years, Miss Osburn remained as Lady Superintendent of Sydney Infirmary for 18 years, returning to London on the Australia in 1885. It was an appropriately named vessel, as Lucy was known to say she felt like an Australian. Before venturing on the long voyage home, she recuperated in the Blue Mountains to strengthen her health and took a shorter voyage to New Zealand to test her sea legs. She did not cut her ties completely from the busily expanding city of Sydney, for she had become reasonably wealthy, with a sizable share portfolio accrued in the colony.

Many years before, the Nightingale Sisters, at the end of their three-year contract, had resigned or been dismissed.

> The later careers of the five nurses who accompanied Lucy Osburn to Sydney largely indicated her judgement confirmed the extreme difficulty they posed to any manager.
>
> *(Gooden, page 313)*

Mary Barker returned to St Thomas' Hospital in May 1874. In 1875 she became Night Superintendent of Edinburgh's Royal Infirmary, then Matron of the Infirmary's Convalescent Hospital. She was forced to resign in 1881 because of complaints against her. In 1889, she became an in-patient of the Prestwich Mental Asylum.

Eliza Blundell became Matron of the NSW Benevolent Society's Asylum where she remained for 23 years. She was known to be a 'complete martinet' and 'harangued her patients'. In 1878 with

Dr Arthur Renwick they formed a training school for nurses and midwives. She remarried, becoming Mrs Elric. She resigned in 1894. Her successor was Rebecca MacKay who had succeeded Lucy Osburn in 1885.

Bessie Chant married William Simpson in 1871. Following his death in 1881, she became Matron of the Gladesville Asylum for the Insane remaining for 26 years. She died of dysentery in 1920 aged 83 years.

Annie Miller went to Brisbane Hospital then to Melbourne. There she took a position at the Hospital for the Insane at Goodna (Victoria) and died in the Melbourne Benevolent Society Asylum in 1907.

Haldane Turiff became Matron of the Alfred Hospital, Melbourne. In 1876 she was investigated three times but cleared of charges of unpleasantness, irritability, having a violent temper, upsetting medical officers and spreading false rumours. She married William Murray in 1880. She was widowed in 1888 and returned to Scotland where she died in 1922.

The relationship between Lucy and Florence Nightingale had deteriorated. Lucy's frankness, conveyed in lengthy letters about problems in Sydney, seemed to have resulted in Miss Nightingale's impatience and annoyance with her envoy.

In 1891, six years after her return to her homeland, Miss Osburn died at the age of 55.

23

An End and a Beginning

17 OCTOBER 1953

The clock on the operating theatre wall surely senses my constant check on its progress, by stubbornly slowing down the mechanism. The black hands are glued together over the number five, and in a little over half an hour this shift and the four years will come to a close. My suitcases are packed in readiness for boarding the North Coast Express tomorrow: goodbye to the Virgin's Retreat.

It is Saturday and so no operation lists are pinned to the theatre noticeboard: the weekends afford an opportunity to catch up on cleaning and making dressings, and as I unload the last drum from the autoclave the phone sets up a jangling from its position on the wall.

'This is Sister in Casualty, Nurse.' The efficient voice speaks decisively and my heart sinks.

'We will be sending up an urgent case needing surgery, a craniotomy, so set up the theatre in readiness.'

A few more details and instructions are added, before I replace the receiver and check the clock again. The hands have advanced five more minutes. This is a day when my own expectations will come to mind first, selfish or otherwise. William will be waiting, two theatre tickets tucked into his pocket. The musical *South Pacific* is opening tonight, 8 p.m. at the Empire Theatre, and this is to be a celebration of my last day at Sydney Hospital. The neurosurgeon on call, a small, dark, hot-tempered man, is well known for his own demonstrations of how high the cranial brace and bit, used to drill into the skull, can bounce off the terrazzo floor in his theatre. This could be disastrous. I have never seen a craniotomy performed. The staff in the instrument room notified, I begin preparing the operating theatre.

Five minutes to six and I mentally urge the clock onwards. The patient has still not arrived from Casualty and, if they are wheeled in before 6 p.m., I will have to scrub and see the operation through to the finish, possibly taking several hours.

Two minutes to six and just as I have given up hope of being relieved the second Theatre Sister on duty, working until 10 p.m. in the Maitland Theatre, appears in the doorway.

Punctuality, No. 12 and last on the list of Indispensable Qualities Desirable in a Nurse, has been without question, perfected.

I swiftly strip off the theatre garb and toss it, with a feeling of satisfaction, into the laundry trolley. I unpin my diamond ring and slip it onto my finger.

Without the need of an emergency to spur me on I run across the courtyard and no-one shouts 'cease running Nurse and walk'. There is no time now for reflection on the nursing profession and the deeply instilled petticoat tyranny of the past century; such pondering will come much later. The bundy clock clicks and with a speed that surprises me I negotiate my last flight down the grand staircase of the Nightingale Wing, the separate quarters that were so important in lifting the nurses' status when it was built in 1869.

I don't look back but keep my eyes focused straight ahead. William is waiting near a corner of the sandstone building opposite the fountain. His face is beaming and he lifts his hat in greeting, as always.

'You've made it through to the end. How does that feel now?'

'Now? It was fun—looking at it from this end,' I reply.

Epilogue

5 November 1953

Two days into our honeymoon we return briefly to Sydney Hospital so that I can take part in the graduation ceremony. The pale blue boardroom, decorated with large bowls of flowers, is a fitting and cheerful background as the room fills with close relatives and friends. The graduates are dressed in nurses' uniform but the cap that designates the year of training is replaced by a veil, a symbolic gesture of our new title, Sister.

The combined May and October finals are represented by 27 graduates. This number includes five of our original group. Barbara with her fragile persona, whom in the beginning I suspected might not last the four years of training, has proved me wrong. Each one receives her diploma, blue bound in book style and a Sydney Hospital badge made of sterling silver, presented by the Vice-President of the National Council for Women. Second prize awarded for my place in the May Finals is a thick biography of Florence Nightingale. Her memory is embraced while we follow Matron Pidgeon's lead and recite the Florence Nightingale pledge, a ritual that reminds me of school assembly—a natural comparison because we are graduates of the School of Nursing.

The press attends and the occasion makes a full-page spread the following day in two newspapers, including a separate image in both editions portraying William at my side proudly holding the diploma. We are singled out because being newly into a honeymoon seems to be a novelty.

The true honeymoon begins the following day as we fly out to spend two weeks on Norfolk Island and on our return the last celebration associated with memories of Sydney Hospital is held at the Pickwick Club. A graduation ball commemorated over a magnum of champagne is the close of a phase in the lives of the friends and their partners, who are all moving towards marriage.

When compared with a lifetime it is a fleeting period, sharing rooms and problems, borrowing each other's clothes, lending a sympathetic ear—four years 'living in' forges friendships that endure for decades.

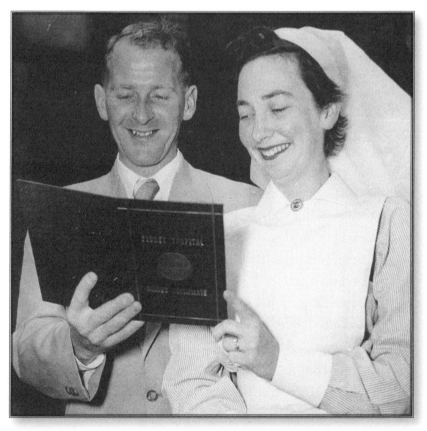

Graduation Day, 1953. (Courtesy Daily Telegraph, 5 November 1953)

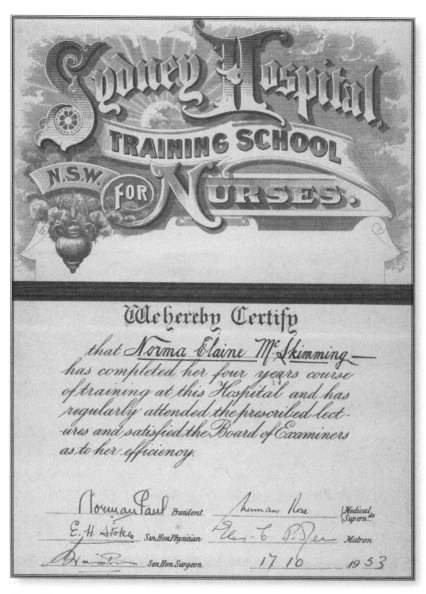

Norma Sim's nurse training certificate.

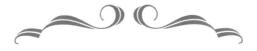

The Nurse's 'If'

If you can grin and joke when all about you
    Are so fed up they don't know what to do,
If you can come on duty and be cheerful,
    When you feel you are on the verge of having' flu,
If you can live the whole day thru' without a wardsmaid
    Admissions pouring in and dinners late,
If you can scrub and comb them all and like it
    And come up smiling when it's half past eight,
If you can think the sister really loves you
    And only runs you round for your own good,
When she tells you that the bathroom is disgraceful
    And your washers never look the way they should,
If you can scrub out everlasting lockers
    Till your knees are red with kneeling on the floor,
And still believe you've joined a noble calling,
    And never long to be at home once more,
If you on junior work can keep the brasses
    So bright they gleam like stars from overhead,

With only one small tin of Brasso polish
That the wardsmaid pinches while you're still in bed,
If you can slog the whole day thru' and never grumble,
If you only seem to polish and wash paint,
If you can do all this and keep your reason,
You're not a nurse, my girl — you're just a Saint!

Author unknown, based on If by Rudyard Kipling

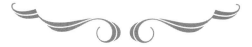

Bibliography

Annual Reports, Sydney Hospital, 1949–50, 1950–51, 1951–52, 1952–53

Brodsky, Isadore, *Sydney's Nurse Crusaders*, Old Sydney Free Press, Sydney, 1968

Doherty, Sirl and Ring (eds), *Modern Practical Nursing Procedures*, Dymocks, Sydney, 1951

Godden, Judith, *Lucy Osburn, A Lady Displaced: Florence Nightingale's envoy to Australia*, Sydney University Press, Sydney, 2006

Lambert, Lionel, 'Macquarie Street buildings', *Centenary Illustrated Sydney Hospital Gazette*, internal hospital publication, Sydney, 1994

McDonnell, Freda, *Miss Nightingale's Young Ladies*, Angus and Robertson, Sydney, 1970

Pitt, Rosemary, 'The Nightingale Nurses in Colonial New South Wales' in *Journal of the Royal Australian Historical Society*, vol. 78, parts 3 and 4, pp. 19–38, December 1992

Wilkinson, Caroline, *Australia's First Hospital: the first 100 years*, self-published, 2005

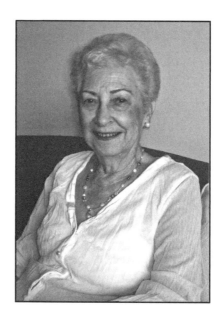

Norma Sim was born in Dorrigo, NSW. In 1953 she graduated from Sydney Hospital Nursing School. She ran her own convalescent home for nine years and then nursed in the public and private hospital systems for more than 20 years. She has traveled extensively and, on her retirement, returned to her childhood love of writing. *Apprentice in Black Stockings* is her fifth book. Her other books include *Diligence and Dairies* (1999), *Sea Poem* (2002), *The Dorrigo Ladies* (1998), and *The Sixty Miler* (2005). She lives on Sydney's North Shore.

First published in Australia in 2010 by
New Holland Publishers (Australia) Pty Ltd
Sydney • Auckland • London • Cape Town

www.newholland.com.au

1/66 Gibbes Street Chatswood NSW 2067 Australia
218 Lake Road Northcote Auckland New Zealand
86 Edgware Road London W2 2EA United Kingdom
80 McKenzie Street Cape Town 8001 South Africa

Copyright © 2010 in text: Norma Sim
Copyright © 2010 in images: various
Copyright © 2010 New Holland Publishers (Australia) Pty Ltd

All rights reserved. No part of this publication may be reproduced, stored in a retrieval system or transmitted, in any form or by any means, electronic, mechanical, photocopying, recording or otherwise, without the prior written permission of the publishers and copyright holders.

National Library of Australia Cataloguing-in-Publication Data:
　Sim, Norma

　　Apprentice in black stockings: recollections of nurse training 1949–1953 / Norma Sim

　　ISBN 9781741109634

　　Sim, Norma.
　　Osburn, Lucy, 1835–1891
　　Sydney Hospital — History — .
　　Nurses — New South Wales — Sydney.
　　Nursing — New South Wales — Sydney
　　History

　　610.73069099441

Publisher: Fiona Schultz
Publishing manager: Lliane Clarke
Senior project editor: Julia Collingwood
Editor: Meryl Potter
Proofreader: Catherine Etteridge
Designer: Tania Gomes
Cover design: Tania Gomes
Production manager: Olga Dementiev
Printer: McPherson's Printing Group, Maryborough, Victoria